Direct Diagnosis in Radiology

Gastrointestinal Imaging

Hans-Juergen Brambs, MD

Professor of Radiology
Chief of the Department of Diagnostic and Interventional Radiology
University Hospital of Ulm
Ulm, Germany

256 Illustrations

Thieme
Stuttgart · New York

Library of Congress
Cataloging-in-Publication Data

Brambs, Hans-Juergen.
   [Gastrointestinales system. English]
   Gastrointestinal imaging / Hans-Juergen
   Brambs ; [translator, John Grossman].
      p. ; cm. – (Direct diagnosis in radiology)
   Includes bibliographical references
   and index.
   ISBN 978-3-13-145101-9
   (TPS, rest of World : alk. paper) –
   ISBN 978-1-60406-040-9
   (TPN, the Americas : alk. paper)
1. Gastrointestinal system–Imaging–
Handbooks, manuals, etc. 2. Gastrointestinal
system–Diseases–Diagnosis–Handbooks,
manuals, etc. I. Title. II. Series.
   [DNLM: 1. Digestive System–radiography–
Handbooks. 2. Diagnosis, Differential–Hand-
books. 3. Digestive System–ultrasonography–
Handbooks. 4. Gastrointestinal Diseases–
diagnosis–Handbooks. WI 39 B815g 2008a]
   RC804.D52B7313 2008
   616.3'307572–dc22   2007039024

This book is an authorized and revised trans-
lation of the German edition published and
copyrighted 2007 by Georg Thieme Verlag,
Stuttgart, Germany. Title of the German
edition: Pareto-Reihe Radiologie:
Gastrointestinales System.

Translator: John Grossman, Schrepkow,
Germany

© 2008 Georg Thieme Verlag KG
Rüdigerstrasse 14, 70469 Stuttgart, Germany
http://www.thieme.de
Thieme New York, 333 Seventh Avenue,
New York, NY 10001, USA
http://www.thieme.com

Cover design: Thieme Publishing Group
Typesetting by Ziegler + Müller,
Kirchentellinsfurt, Germany
Printed by APPL, aprinta Druck,
Wemding, Germany

ISBN 978-3-13-145101-9
(TPS, Rest of World)
ISBN 978-1-60406-040-9
(TPN, The Americas)
                              1 2 3 4 5 6

Important note: Medicine is an ever-chang-
ing science undergoing continual development. Research and clinical experience are
continually expanding our knowledge, in particular our knowledge of proper treatment
and drug therapy. Insofar as this book men-
tions any dosage or application, readers may
rest assured that the authors, editors, and
publishers have made every effort to ensure
that such references are in accordance with
**the state of knowledge at the time of pro-
duction of the book.**

Nevertheless, this does not involve, imply, or
express any guarantee or responsibility on
the part of the publishers in respect to any
dosage instructions and forms of applications
stated in the book. **Every user is requested to
examine carefully** the manufacturers' leaf-
lets accompanying each drug and to check, if
necessary in consultation with a physician or
specialist, whether the dosage schedules
mentioned therein or the contraindications
stated by the manufacturers differ from the
statements made in the present book. Such
examination is particularly important with
drugs that are either rarely used or have been
newly released on the market. Every dosage
schedule or every form of application used is
entirely at the user's own risk and responsibility. The authors and publishers request every
user to report to the publishers any discrepan-
cies or inaccuracies noticed. If errors in this
work are found after publication, errata will
be posted at www.thieme.com on the product
description page.

To my sons Benedikt, Florian, and Sebastian.

Contents

5 Esophagus

6 Stomach and Duodenum

7 Small Bowel

8 Colon and Anus

9 Abdominal Cavity

AFP	Alpha-fetoprotein
AIDS	Acquired immuno-deficiency syndrome
ASA	Aminosalicylic acid
CO₂	Carbon dioxide
COPD	Chronic obstructive pulmonary disease
CRP	C-reactive protein
CT	Computed tomography, computed tomogram
DD	Differential diagnosis
DAS	Digital subtraction angiography
ERCP	Endoscopic retrograde cholangiopancreatography
FDG	18F-Fluorodeoxyglucose
FNH	Focal nodular hyperplasia
FSE	Fast spin echo
GE	Gradient echo
GIST	Gastrointestinal stromal tumor
HASTE	Half Fourier single shot turbo spin echo
HCC	Hepatocellular carcinoma
HU	Hounsfield unit
HELLP	Hemolysis, elevated liver enzymes, low platelet count
HIV	Human immunodeficiency virus
IPMN	Intraductal papillary mucinous neoplasm
LDH	Lactate dehydrogenase
MDCT	Multi-detector CT
MIP	Maximum intensity projection
MRC	MR cholangiography
MRCP	MR cholangio-pancreatography
MRI	Magnetic resonance imaging
NSAID	Nonsteroidal anti-inflammatory drugs
PAS	Paraaminosalicylic acid
PET	Positron emission tomography
PSC	Primary sclerosing cholangitis
PTC	Percutaneous transhepatic cholangiography
RARE	Rapid acquisition with relaxation enhancement
RES	Reticuloendothelial system
RI	Resistive index
SPIO	Superparamagnetic iron oxide
TACE	Transarterial chemoembolization
TAE	Transarterial embolization
TIPS	Transjugular intrahepatic portosystemic shunt
VIBE	Volume interpolated breath-hold examination
WHO	World Health Organization

Definition

Chronic liver disease with destruction of the lobar architecture • Proliferation of connective tissue • Regeneration nodules and necrosis.

► **Epidemiology**
More common in men • Usually occurs in middle-aged and older people.

► **Etiology, pathophysiology, pathogenesis**
Most often caused by chronic alcohol abuse and viral hepatitis • Less common causes include chronic cholestasis, autoimmune disorders, impaired hepatic venous blood flow (Budd–Chiari syndrome), and metabolic disorders (α1-antitrypsin deficiency, hemochromatosis, Wilson disease, glycogenosis).

Imaging Signs

► **Modality of choice**
Ultrasound, CT.

► **Pathognomonic findings**
The liver is either enlarged or reduced in size • Hypertrophic caudate lobe • Irregular nodular contour • Nodular structure (micronodular form is more common in alcoholic liver disease, macronodular form in hepatitis B) • Compression of the intrahepatic veins and portal vein feeders • Dilated portal and splenic veins • Splenomegaly • *Complications:* Portal hypertension (varices in the abdominal cavity and esophagus, recanalization of the umbilical vein) • Ascites • HCC.

► **Ultrasound findings**
Primary modality in cirrhosis; ultrasound in combination with measurement of AFP is a screening procedure for HCC • Irregular nodular contour • Deformed organ • Mixed hypoechoic and hyperechoic parenchymal structure • Color Doppler studies show a prominent hepatic artery with increased blood flow • Direction of flow in the portal vein is reversed.

► **CT findings**
In early forms, CT findings are normal in 25% of cases • Irregular nodular contour • Heterogeneous parenchyma with nodules of varying size • Nodules with increased iron content can appear hyperdense • Heterogeneous contrast enhancement.

► **MRI findings**
T1-weighted images show hypointense fibrotic changes (expanded periportal field and netlike structures) very early • On T2-weighted images, the inflammatory fibrotic tissue usually appears as increased signal • Regenerating nodules on T1-weighted images are hypointense to hyperintense, on T2-weighted images isointense to hypointense • After contrast administration they appear hypointense to adjacent liver tissue • Dysplastic nodules are often hyperintense on T1-weighted images and hypointense on T2-weighted images • Heterogeneous pattern of enhancement after contrast administration • Smaller nodules (<20 mm) are seen exclusively in the early arterial phase (prevalence is about 30%); they usually represent arterioportal shunts and regenerating nodules (however, less than 10% represent HCC) • With SPIO, the fibrotic ligaments are

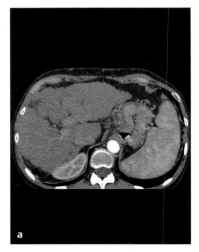 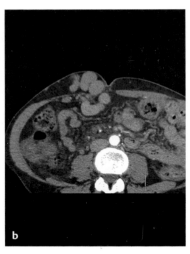

Fig. 1.1 a, b Cirrhosis of the liver. CT, early arterial phase.
a Enlarged liver with irregular nodular contour and splenomegaly.
b Massive venous varices in the abdominal wall with patent umbilical vein.

often more readily identifiable; these remain hyperintense on T2-weighted images • Hepatocellular carcinoma is best demonstrated on double contrast studies (gadolinium and SPIO) • Indications for double contrast technique include preoperative studies for liver transplantation.

Clinical Aspects

▶ **Typical presentation**
Symptoms may be uncharacteristic • Fatigue • Weight loss • Jaundice • Hard liver • Splenomegaly • Spider nevi • Petechial hemorrhages • Gynecomastia • Encephalopathy.

▶ **Therapeutic options**
Treatment of the underlying disorder • Elimination of the noxious agents • Liver transplantation.

▶ **Course and prognosis**
This depends on the pathogenesis of the cirrhosis, the severity of the loss of liver function, and the patient's lifestyle (for example, abstinence from alcohol) • 1-year mortality in type A cirrhosis (Child's classification) is slight, in type B 30%, and in type C 50%.

▶ **What does the clinician want to know?**
Severity of the complications (ascites and varices) • Development of HCC.

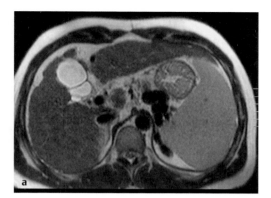

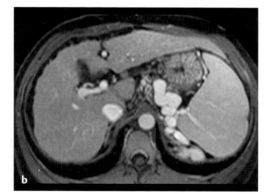

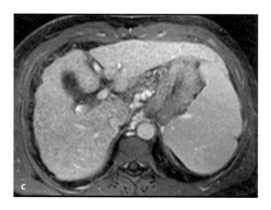

Fig. 1.2 a–c   Cirrhosis of the liver. **a** T2-weighted MR image. Slightly irregular and nodular liver contour, splenomegaly, and splenic varices. **b** T1-weighted MR image after contrast administration, arterial phase. Pronounced splenic varices. **c** T1-weighted image after contrast administration, late portal venous phase. Irregular nodular surface with patchy parenchyma from regenerating nodules. Dilated coronary veins and esophageal veins.

Differential Diagnosis

Budd–Chiari syndrome	– Occluded hepatic veins
	– Nodular enhancement pattern after contrast administration
Diffuse metastases	– Normal sized caudate lobe
	– No atrophic segments
	– No collateral vessels

Tips and Pitfalls

Regenerating nodules or dysplastic nodules may be mistaken for HCC.

Selected Literature

Danet IM et al. MR imaging of diffuse liver disease. Radiol Clin North Am 2003; 41: 67–87

Dodd GD et al. Spectrum of imaging findings of the liver in end-stage cirrhosis: Part I, gross morphology and diffuse abnormalities. AJR 1999; 173: 1031–1036

Holland AE et al. Importance of small (< 20 mm) enhancing lesions seen only during the hepatic arterial phase at MR imaging of the cirrhotic liver: evaluation and comparison with the whole explanted liver. Radiology 2005; 237: 938–944

Definition

Isolated or multiple fluid-filled masses in the hepatic parenchyma.

▶ **Epidemiology**
   Prevalence in healthy liver is 2–7% • Incidence is greater in elderly people • More common in women • Autosomal dominant polycystic disease is associated with multiple hepatic cysts in 40% of cases.

▶ **Etiology, pathophysiology, pathogenesis**
   Developmental anomalies that do not communicate with the biliary system.

Imaging Signs

▶ **Modality of choice**
   Ultrasound, MRI.

▶ **Pathognomonic findings**
   Isolated or multiple fluid-filled cavities of varying size • Surrounded by a thin capsule • Sharply demarcated from the parenchyma • The thin wall does not enhance with contrast • Liver is enlarged (in polycystic disease).

▶ **Ultrasound findings**
   Anechoic spherical masses with marked acoustic enhancement.

▶ **MRI findings**
   Hypointense on T1-weighted images and hyperintense on T2-weighted images • Hyperintense on T1-weighted images after hemorrhage • Infected cysts show thickening and enhancement of the cyst wall.

▶ **CT findings**
   Cysts are hypodense on unenhanced scans with density values equivalent to water (0–10 HU) • Hemorrhage appears hyperdense on unenhanced scans • Discrete calcifications are occasionally seen in the cyst wall • The cyst wall or surrounding tissue does not enhance with contrast unless the cyst is infected.

Clinical Aspects

▶ **Typical presentation**
   Asymptomatic • Incidental finding • Large solitary cysts and polycystic renal disease are associated with hepatomegaly.

▶ **Therapeutic options**
   Isolated hepatic cysts do not require treatment • Large cysts may require surgical fenestration • Percutaneous aspiration and sclerotherapy are rarely indicated.

▶ **Course and prognosis**
   In polycystic disease, hepatic cysts can bleed, become infected, or rupture.

▶ **What does the clinician want to know?**
   Exclude cystic metastases and abscesses. Complication due to hemorrhage or infection.

Fig. 1.3 Polycystic liver. Ultrasound. Multiple large anechoic masses.

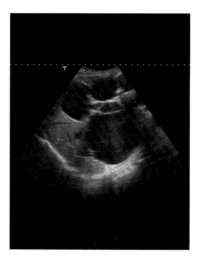

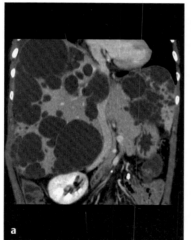

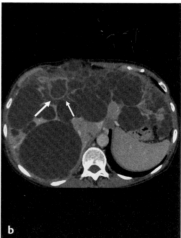

Fig. 1.4 a, b Polycystic liver and spleen. CT (**a**). Infected cyst with thickened wall showing marked enhancement (arrows; **b**).

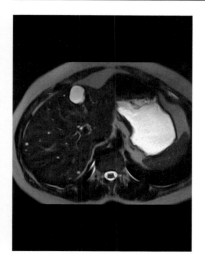

Fig. 1.5 Hepatic cysts. T2-weighted MR image. Multiple, mostly small hepatic cysts.

Differential Diagnosis

Abscess	– Thick, enhancing capsule – Fever
Echinococcus cyst	– Calcifications in the capsule – Evidence of a floating membrane with ruptured lamellae
Cystadenoma	– Septated tumor
Cystic, necrotising	– Often with areas of solid tissue showing variable enhancement
Metastases	– Central or ring enhancement – Metastases of cystic tumors are often indistinguishable

Tips and Pitfalls

Misinterpretation of a cyst as a metastasis or abscess.

Selected Literature

Brancatelli G et al. Fibropolycystic liver disease: CT and MR imaging findings. Radio-Graphics 2005; 25: 659–670

Mathieu D et al. Benign liver tumors. Magn Reson Imaging Clin North Am 1997; 5: 255–288

Mortele KJ et al. Cystic focal liver lesions in the adult: differential CT and MR imaging features. Radiographics 2001; 21: 895–910

Liver

Definition

Benign malformations of the biliary system.

▶ **Epidemiology**
Prevalence is 1–3%.

▶ **Etiology, pathophysiology, pathogenesis**
Presumably a malformation with proliferation of bile ducts (cystic dilated bile ducts occasionally containing amorphous material) • Lesion is lined with cuboidal epithelium • Embedded in fibrous stroma • There is no communication with the bile ducts • Macroscopically the lesion appears as a whitish-gray nodule.

Imaging Signs

▶ **Modality of choice**
Ultrasound, MRI.

▶ **Pathognomonic findings**
CT and MRI show multiple disseminated small nodules (0.5–1.5 cm) • Isolated lesions are rare • Nodules usually occur in the subcapsular region • MRI findings differ from ultrasound—MRI shows multiple small cysts that are not detected in the ultrasound scan • Lesions usually do not enhance (where the cystic component predominates) • Lesions enhance only in the rare cases where the solid component predominates • Follow-up examinations demonstrate no change in the number or size of the lesions.

▶ **MRI findings**
Well demarcated • Slightly hypointense on T1-weighted images and hyperintense on T2-weighted images (less so than cysts) • After contrast administration, the lesion shows ring enhancement in every phase • MR cholangiography shows cystic changes that do not communicate with the biliary system.

▶ **Ultrasound findings**
Hepatic parenchyma exhibits heterogeneous structure • Small hypoechoic to hyperechoic nodules are present.

▶ **CT findings**
Hypodense nodules are present, which are better demarcated from the surrounding liver tissue after contrast administration.

Clinical Aspects

▶ **Typical presentation**
Clinically asymptomatic • Usually an incidental finding • No abnormal laboratory findings.

▶ **Therapeutic options**
None.

▶ **Course and prognosis**
A few cases of malignant transformation have been described.

▶ **What does the clinician want to know?**
Exclude metastases.

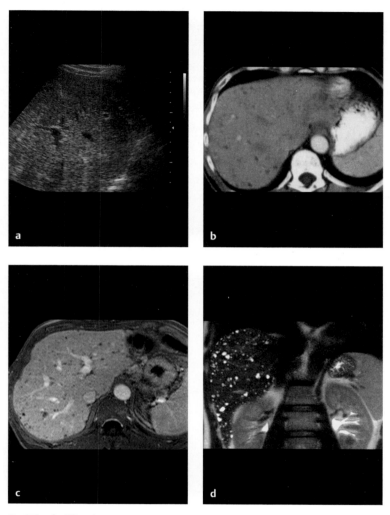

Fig. 1.6a–d   Biliary hamartomas.
a Ultrasound. Inhomogeneous image showing small, ill-defined hypoechoic focal lesions.
b CT after contrast administration. Multiple small hypodense areas that do not enhance.
c MR image after contrast administration. Multiple small hypointense focal lesions that do not enhance.
d MR image, HASTE. Multiple hyperintense focal lesions with a cystic appearance.

Differential Diagnosis

Hepatic cysts	– Recognizable as such, especially on ultrasound
	– Often larger than 1.5 cm
Caroli syndrome	– Communication with the biliary system
	– Often larger cystic dilations
	– With concretions and a tendency to become infected
Metastases	– Rarely purely cystic (except for gastrointestinal stromal tumors)
	– Enhancement depends on the primary tumor

Tips and Pitfalls

Lesions can be confused with metastases, both on diagnostic images and at laparoscopy or open surgery.

Selected Literature

Lev-Toaff AS et al. The radiologic and pathologic spectrum of biliary hamartomas. AJR 1995; 165: 309–313

Semelka RC et al. Biliary hamartomas: solitary and multiple lesions shown on current MR techniques including gadolinium enhancement. J Magn Reson Imaging 1999; 10: 196–201

Zheng RQ et al. Imaging findings of biliary hamartomas. World J Gastroenterol 2005; 13: 6354–6359

Definition

Isolated or multiple accumulations of pus in the hepatic parenchyma.

▶ **Epidemiology**
   Certain forms such as amebic abscess are endemic in Africa, southeast Asia, and Latin America.

▶ **Etiology, pathophysiology, pathogenesis**
   In 20–40% of cases, no cause can be identified • The most common identifiable cause is biliary tract infection with stones or other obstructive disorders • Less often ascending abdominal infections (appendicitis, diverticulitis, inflammatory bowel disease) • Secondary to interventions such as radiofrequency ablation (< 2%) and transarterial chemoembolization • Immunosuppressed patients are at increased risk • Usually the abscess contains a mixture of pathogens.

Imaging Signs

▶ **Modality of choice**
   Ultrasound, CT.

▶ **Pathognomonic findings**
   Multiple small lesions or isolated large lesions • Large quantities of debris present initially • Contents liquefy as the lesion matures • Lesion is surrounded by an enhancing halo of variable width • Appearance depends on the pathogen—for example, *Candida* produces multiple small abscesses (< 5 mm).

▶ **Ultrasound findings**
   Usually hypoechoic to anechoic round mass • Can also appear hyperechoic prior to liquefaction • Occasionally an irregular wall is detectable • Occasionally appears septated and contains debris • Gas appears highly echodense with an acoustic shadow.

▶ **CT findings**
   Hypodense on unenhanced scans • An enhancing halo of varying width appears after contrast administration • In small *Candida* abscesses, the arterial phase demonstrates more lesions than the portal venous phase.

▶ **MRI findings**
   Very low signal intensity on T1-weighted images and very high intensity on T2-weighted images • Enhancing capsule of varying thickness • MRCP can demonstrate biliary causes.

Clinical Aspects

▶ **Typical presentation**
   Onset of pyogenic liver abscess is usually insidious, with fever and pain in the right upper abdomen • Acute symptoms are more common in amebic abscess • Hepatomegaly • Tenderness over the liver.

▶ **Therapeutic options**
   Aspiration and drainage • Treatment of the underlying disorder in abscesses due to biliary causes.

Fig. 1.7 Liver abscess. Ultrasound. Inhomogeneous hypoechoic liver mass in an incompletely liquefied liver abscess.

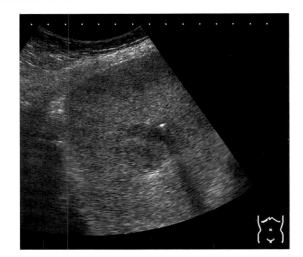

Fig. 1.8 Liver abscess. CT. Confluent hypodense areas in an incompletely liquefied liver abscess.

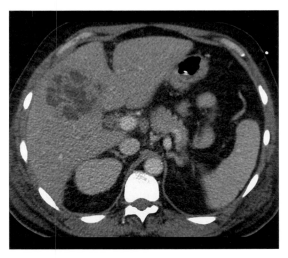

▶ **Course and prognosis**
Healing is usually possible with adequate drainage and elimination of the underlying cause ● Mortality is 8% ● Fungal infections and malignant processes have a
poorer prognosis ● Surgery is now rarely indicated.

▶ **What does the clinician want to know?**
Early detection of an abscess ● Identification of the underlying disorder.

Differential Diagnosis

Cyst	– No enhancing capsule
	– No fever
Echinococcus cyst	– Calcifications in the capsule
	– Evidence of a floating membrane with ruptured lamellae
Cystadenoma	– Septated tumor
	– No fever
	– Rare
Cystic, necrotising	– Often with areas of solid tissue showing variable enhancement
Metastases	– No fever
	– Small metastases showing ring enhancement are morphologically indistinguishable

Tips and Pitfalls

Can be misinterpreted as a normal cyst, tumor with cystic degeneration, or metastases.

Selected Literature

Balci NC et al. MR imaging of infected liver lesions. Magn Reson Imaging Clin North Am
2002; 10: 121–135

Giorgio A et al. Pyogenic liver abscesses: 13 years of experience in percutaneous needle
aspiration with ultrasound guidance. Radiology 1995; 195: 122–124

Metser U et al. Fungal liver infection in immunocompromised patients: depiction with
multiphasic contrast-enhanced helical CT. Radiology 2005; 235: 97–105

Definition

Parasitic infection with *Echinococcus granulosus*.

▶ **Epidemiology**

Endemic in sheep and cattle raising areas • Sheep and cattle are intermediate hosts.

▶ **Etiology, pathophysiology, pathogenesis**

Infection by the dog tapeworm in the larval stage • Infection occurs by direct contact with the final host (dog) or via contaminated water or food • The embryos migrate through the intestinal mucosa and reach the liver via the portal vein, where they initially form small cysts that grow 2–3 cm per year • The liver and lung are the most common sites of infection.

Imaging Signs

▶ **Modality of choice**

Ultrasound, CT.

▶ **Pathognomonic findings**

Small hydatid cysts appear identical to common cysts • Larger cysts form daughter cysts and membranes that can slough off or rupture • Findings may include "hydatid sand" when scolices are shed from the inner layer • Calcifications may occur in the outer layer in the late stages of the disease.

▶ **Ultrasound findings**

Anechoic cysts with membranes that can undulate with motion • Calcifications • Intact capsules may appear as a double line (ectocyst and endocyst).

▶ **CT findings**

Cyst with daughter cysts, membranes, and calcifications.

▶ **MRI findings**

T1-weighted and T2-weighted images show a pericystic "rim sign" of low signal intensity • T1-weighted and T2-weighted images show hypointense floating membranes • Hyperintense cysts with membranes are visualized on T2-weighted images • Calcifications are often impossible to detect in fibrous tissue.

▶ **Direct cystographic findings**

Cystic mass, occasionally communicating with the biliary system.

Clinical Aspects

▶ **Typical presentation**

Often an asymptomatic incidental finding • Occasionally there is a sensation of pressure in the upper abdomen • Most severe complication is anaphylactic shock • *Echinococcus* titer is very reliable in liver involvement.

▶ **Therapeutic options**

Surgical excision with irrigation of the cyst cavity • Aspiration and drainage should be used with caution because of the risk of anaphylactic shock • Medical treatment is with mebendazole.

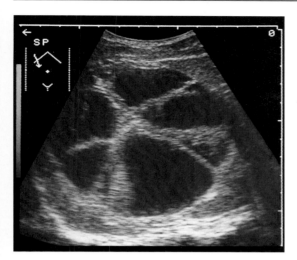

Fig. 1.9 Hydatid disease (cystic echinococcosis). Ultrasound. Hydatid cyst with spokelike septa.

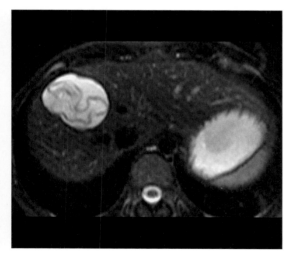

Fig. 1.10 Hydatid disease. T2-weighted MR image. The sloughed membrane of the hydatid cyst is clearly seen.

▶ **Course and prognosis**

Poor prognosis ● Less than 20% of cases are resectable ● Most severe complication is rupture of a cyst in the abdominal cavity.

▶ **What does the clinician want to know?**

Exclude a common cyst.

Differential Diagnosis

Simple cysts	– No membranes and usually homogeneous fluid
	– No calcifications
Cystic tumors	– Usually a thicker wall that enhances with contrast
Metastases of cystic tumors	– Usually smaller and multiple

Tips and Pitfalls

Aspiration without obtaining a titer ● Irrigating with alcohol or silver nitrate solution without excluding a rare communication between the cyst and the biliary system.

Selected Literature

Czermak BV et al. Echinococcus granulosus revisited: radiologic patterns seen in pediatric and adult patients. AJR 2001; 177: 1051–1056

Oto A et al. Focal inflammatory diseases of the liver. Eur J Radiol 1999; 32: 61–75

Pedrosa I et al. Hydatid disease: Radiologic and pathologic features and complications. RadioGraphics 2000; 20: 795–817

Definition

Parasitic infection with *Echinococcus multilocularis.*

▶ **Epidemiology**
Endemic in central Europe (southwestern Germany, Austria, Switzerland, and northeastern France), the American Midwest, Alaska, Canada, and parts of the Russia ● Wild rodents are intermediate hosts.

▶ **Etiology, pathophysiology, pathogenesis**
Infection by the fox tapeworm in the larval stage ● Infection occurs by contact with the final host (usually fox, less often cat or dog) or via contaminated water or food ● The embryos migrate through the intestinal mucosa and reach the liver via the portal vein or lymph vessels, where they form small cysts that grow (3–20 mm) ● Infiltrative spread ● The liver and lung are the most common sites of infection.

Imaging Signs

▶ **Modality of choice**
Ultrasound, CT.

▶ **Pathognomonic findings**
Solid, infiltrating mass ● Half of all cases show spread within the hilum of the liver with dilatation of the intrahepatic bile ducts and infiltration of the portal vein (which occasionally leads to reduced perfusion and atrophy) ● Large lesions show central necrosis ● Amorphous calcifications occur in the late stage.

▶ **Ultrasound findings**
Isolated or multiple ill-defined hyperechoic masses ("hailstorm" sign) with calcifications ● Large lesions show central hypoechoic areas (necrosis).

▶ **CT findings**
Hypodense mass resembling a tumor or metastasis ● Enhances slightly with contrast ● Small cysts or discrete eggshell calcifications of the septa may be detectable on high-resolution images.

▶ **MRI findings**
T2-weighted images show solid components and multiple small cysts or larger irregular cysts ● Central necrosis in large lesions appears hyperintense on T2-weighted images ● Calcifications have low signal intensity ● Slight enhancement after contrast administration ● MRCP demonstrates stenosis of the central bile ducts.

▶ **PET findings**
This is the only imaging modality that can assess viability ● Shows response to treatment ● Suitable for demonstrating recurrent lesions and "metastases."

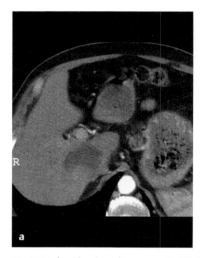 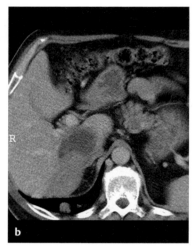

Fig. 1.11 a, b Alveolar echinococcosis. CT after contrast administration. Alveolar echinococcosis with partially cystic and partially tumorlike pattern of involvement in the early arterial phase (**a**) and venous phase (**b**).

Clinical Aspects

▶ **Typical presentation**
   Unspecific abdominal pain ● Weight loss ● Fatigue ● Jaundice ● *Echinococcus* titer is very reliable in liver involvement.
▶ **Therapeutic options**
   Resection and transplantation ● Medical treatment is with mebendazole.
▶ **Course and prognosis**
   Poor prognosis ● Usually not resectable at the time of the diagnosis.
▶ **What does the clinician want to know?**
   Exclude malignant tumors ● Are lesions resectable?

Differential Diagnosis

Cholangiocarcinoma	– Indentation of the liver capsule is fairly typical – Contrast enhancement is usually late (10 minutes) – Calcifications in 20% of cases
HCC	– Usually in a cirrhotic liver – Hypervascular lesion with rapid washout – AFP is raised
Metastases	– Usually no cholestasis – Confluent metastases of a colorectal carcinoma can appear very similar

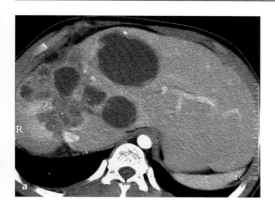

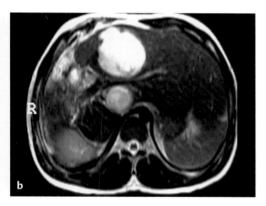

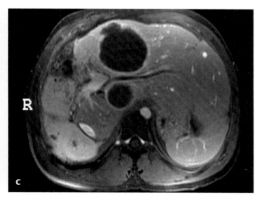

Fig. 1.12 a–c Alveolar echinococcus after liver resection. CT and MR image. Solid and cystic changes in alveolar echinococcus with discrete calcifications that are only detectable on the CT.

Tips and Pitfalls

Can be misinterpreted as a malignant tumor.

Selected Literature

Bresson-Hadni S et al. A twenty-year history of alveolar echinococcosis: analysis of a series of 117 patients from eastern France. Eur J Gastroenterol Hepatol 2000; 12: 327–336

Kodama Y et al. Alveolar echinococcosis: MR findings in the liver. Radiology 2003; 228: 172–174

Reuter S et al. Structured treatment interruption in patients with alveolar echinococcosis. Hepatology 2004; 39: 509–517

Definition

Benign mesenchymal, spongiform tumor of the liver • Spongiform nodule with blood-filled cavities separated from each other by numerous septa • Larger hemangiomas have fibrotic areas.

▶ **Epidemiology**
Occurs sporadically • Often associated with focal nodular hyperplasia • Most common benign tumor of the liver • Occurs in 5–7% of the population • More common in females • Occurs in all age groups • Size ranges from a few millimeters to 20 cm.

Imaging Signs

▶ **Modality of choice**
Ultrasound, MRI

▶ **Pathognomonic findings**
Well-demarcated mass exhibiting a characteristic iris-like pattern of enhancement that persists for a long time due to the slow flow • Small hemangiomas (< 1 cm) can enhance rapidly and briefly (capillary hemangiomas) • Larger hemangiomas may exhibit partial thrombosis and fibrosis) • Calcifications are rare.

▶ **Ultrasound findings**
Well-demarcated, homogeneously hyperechoic mass • Often exhibits slight acoustic enhancement • Power Doppler occasionally shows unspecific flow phenomena.

▶ **MRI findings**
Homogeneously hypointense on T1-weighted images, hyperintense on T2-weighted images (especially in the late T2-weighted phase) • Strong contrast enhancement begins very early peripherally and lesions fill in over time; filling is often complete only in the very late phases • Large hemangiomas may exhibit filling defects • Hypointense in late phases after administration of hepatobiliary contrast agent • Small hemangiomas may enhance rapidly and strongly, but briefly.

▶ **CT findings**
Usually slightly hypodense on unenhanced scans • Contrast behavior is identical to MRI.

▶ **Angiographic findings**
Typical "cotton wool" appearance • No longer used for diagnostic imaging.

Clinical Aspects

▶ **Typical presentation**
Usually an incidental finding • Very large hemangiomas can produce a sensation of pressure • Slightly increased susceptibility to bleeding in trauma.

▶ **Therapeutic options**
Embolization or resection of symptomatic lesions may be indicated.

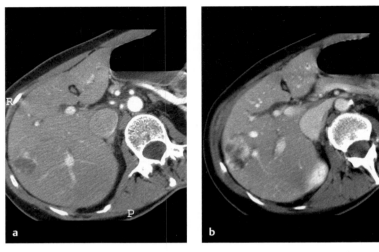

Fig. 1.13 a, b Cavernous hemangioma. CT, early arterial (**a**) and portal venous (**b**) phases. In the early arterial phase, only the periphery of the hemangioma enhances. The portal venous phase shows a nodular pattern of enhancement.

► **Course and prognosis**
  Growth is occasionally observed in larger hemangiomas ● Malignant degeneration does not occur.
► **What does the clinician want to know?**
  Rule out metastases or malignant tumors.

Differential Diagnosis

Focal nodular hyperplasia	– Uptake of hepatobiliary contrast agents in the late phase in MRI
	– Usually not possible in small lesions using CT
Adenoma	– Homogeneous contrast enhancement
	– Not hyperechoic on ultrasound
HCC	– Usually in a cirrhotic liver
	– Rapid passage of contrast agent
	– Not as hyperechoic on ultrasound
	– AFP is raised
Hypervascular metastases	– Usually multiple, smaller focal lesions
	– Usually not hyperechoic on ultrasound

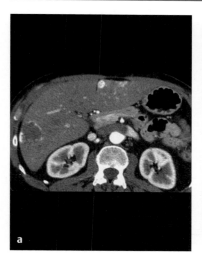
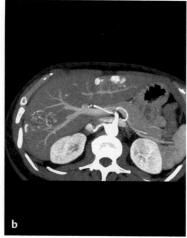

Fig. 1.14a, b Cavernous hemangioma. CT, early arterial phase (**a**) and MIP reconstruction (**b**). The small hemangioma in the left hepatic lobe fills immediately in the arterial phase whereas the larger hemangioma in the right lobe initially shows only peripheral enhancement. In the portal venous phase, the small hemangiomas in the left hepatic lobe are visualized with high contrast while the large hemangioma in the right lobe shows an increasingly strandlike enhancement pattern (**b**).

Tips and Pitfalls

Too many diagnostic studies (ultrasound may be helpful when CT or MRI findings are equivocal, and dynamic MRI including late T2-weighted images may be helpful when CT or ultrasound findings are equivocal).

Selected Literature

Danet IM et al. Giant hemangioma of the liver: MR imaging characteristics in 24 patients. Magn Reson Imaging 2003; 21: 95–101
Kim T et al. Discrimination of small hepatic hemangiomas from hypervascular malignant tumors smaller than 3 cm with three-phase helical CT. Radiology 2001; 219: 699–706
Leslie DF et al. Distinction between cavernous hemangiomas of the liver and hepatic metastases on CT: value of contrast enhancement patterns. AJR 1995; 164: 625–629

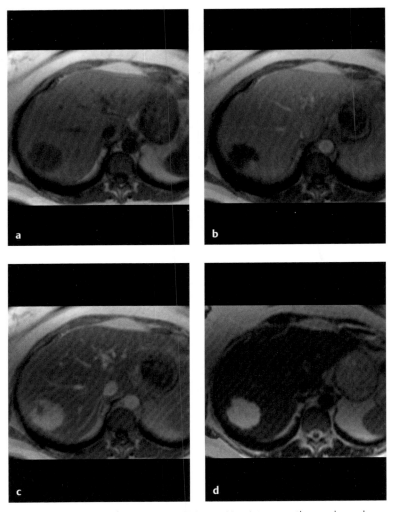

Fig. 1.15 a–d Cavernous hemangioma. MR image. Hypointense on the unenhanced scan (**a**). Partially nodular pattern of peripheral enhancement in the early arterial phase (**b**). Nearly complete enhancement in the late venous phase (**c**). The T2-weighted image shows a relatively homogeneous hyperintense lesion with smooth contours (**d**).

Definition
....

Highly vascularized benign tumor of the liver ● Abnormal nodular internal structure (resembling cirrhotic nodules) with vascular malformations and bile ducts ● Lesions contain varying numbers of Kupffer cells.

► **Epidemiology**

Second most common benign tumor of the liver ● Average patient age is 30–50 years ● Four to eight times more common in women than in men ● Multiple focal nodular hyperplasias and associated hemangiomas can be observed in 20% of cases.

► **Etiology, pathophysiology, pathogenesis**

Presumably a hyperplastic reaction to arterial malformation ● Growth and vascularization may be influenced by female hormones ● Classic tumors occur in 80% of cases; 20% are atypical (usually telangiectatic forms combining genetic and morphologic elements of focal nodular hyperplasia and adenomas).

Imaging Signs
....

► **Modality of choice**

MRI with hepatobiliary contrast agents ● Multiphasic CT.

► **Pathognomonic findings**

Well-demarcated, highly vascularized focal nodular lesion (usually < 5 cm) ● Enhancement after contrast administration is almost exclusively arterial ● Often there will be a stellate "scar." ● The "scar" and the fibrotic strands contain dysplastic arteries and bile ducts.

► **MRI findings**

Isointense to hypointense on T1-weighted images, isointense to hyperintense on T2-weighted images ● The central "scar" is almost invariably hyperintense on T2-weighted images ● Nodular homogeneous contrast enhancement occurs in the arterial phase with rapid passage of the contrast agent ● The "scar" enhances in the later phases ● SPIO is taken up by the reticuloendothelial system (signal is usually not as sharply diminished as in the normal liver ● Hepatobiliary gadolinium compounds also produce pronounced enhancement on late images.

► **CT findings**

On unenhanced scans, lesions appear isodense or slightly hypodense to surrounding liver tissue ● Pronounced nodular contrast enhancement in the arterial phase is followed by rapid passage of contrast agent in later phases ● The central "scar" enhances in the later phases.

► **Ultrasound findings**

Often poorly demarcated ● Usually slightly hyperechoic ● Contrast studies clearly visualize the vascular malformations (resembling spokes of a wheel) and the highly vascular mass, which (in contrast with CT and MRI) shows reperfusion in the portal venous phase.

► **Hepatobiliary sequential scintigraphy**

No longer used.

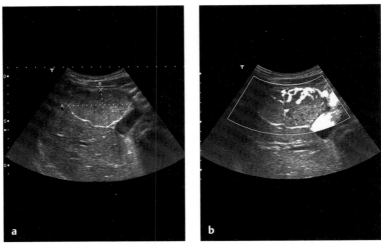

Fig. 1.16 a, b Focal nodular hyperplasia. Ultrasound. Echo texture resembles the liver (**a**). Lesion is bounded by a pseudocapsule. Color Doppler (**b**) demonstrates a spokelike pattern of hypervascularity.

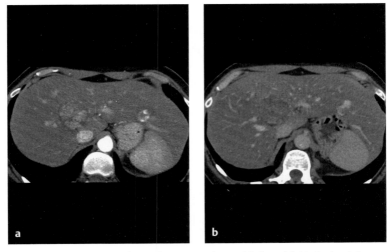

Fig. 1.17 a, b Focal nodular hyperplasia. CT. Early arterial phase (**a**). Marked nodular enhancement. Portal venous phase (**b**). Much less enhancement. A hemangioma is also visualized in the left hepatic lobe.

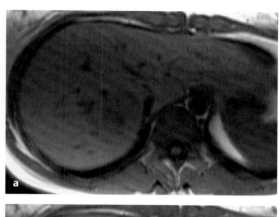

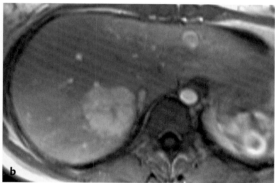

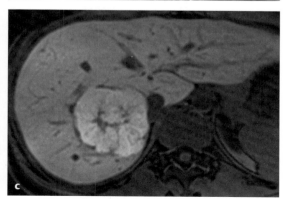

Fig. 1.18 a–c Focal nodular hyperplasia. MRI using a hepatobiliary contrast agent. **a** On unenhanced T1w sequence hypointense lesion within the right liver lobe. **b** Significant contrast enhancement in the early arterial phase. **c** High concentration of the contrast agent in the late phase with good demarcation of the "scar".

Clinical Aspects

▶ **Typical presentation**
Usually an incidental finding ● Large masses can cause a sensation of pressure.

▶ **Therapeutic options**
Hormones should be discontinued ● Large symptomatic masses may require surgical resection or transarterial embolization ● Resection is indicated for atypical focal nodular hyperplasia with a mass that cannot be clearly differentiated from other tumors.

▶ **Course and prognosis**
No malignant degeneration ● Hemorrhages probably occur only in the telangiectatic forms ● Diagnostic aspiration is usually not indicated, given the other available options.

▶ **What does the clinician want to know?**
Rule out other hypervascular tumors or changes.

Differential Diagnosis

Adenoma	– Enhances slightly less
	– No central "scar"
	– No uptake of hepatobiliary gadolinium compounds in the late phase
	– Larger tumors show signs of acute or chronic hemorrhages
Hemangioma	– Iris-like contrast filling
	– High signal intensity on T2-weighted images
	– Very small hemangiomas can have an identical appearance
Fibrolamellar HCC	– Usually large tumors with necrotic areas and calcifications and metastases
	– Contains genuine scars that have lower signal intensity on T2-weighted images and do not enhance
	– No uptake of hepatobiliary gadolinium compounds in the late phase
HCC	– Usually in a cirrhotic liver
	– AFP is raised
	– Hepatobiliary gadolinium compounds are absorbed only in highly differentiated tumors
Hypervascular metastases	– Multiple lesions are usually present
	– Often have ill-defined margins and central necrosis
	– No uptake of hepatobiliary gadolinium compounds in the late phase

Tips and Pitfalls
....

Monophasic examination protocol: The hypervascularity of focal nodular hyperplasia may no longer be detectable in the portal venous phase on MRI and CT.

Selected Literature

Grazioli L et al. Accurate differentiation of focal nodular hyperplasia from hepatic adenoma at gadobenatedimeglumine-enhanced MR imaging: prospective study. Radiology 2005; 236: 166–177

Hussain SM et al. Focal nodular hyperplasia: findings at state-of-the-art MR imaging, US, CT, and pathologic analysis. RadioGraphics 2004; 24: 3–19

Nguyen BN et al. Focal nodular hyperplasia of the liver: a comprehensive pathologic study of 305 lesions and recognition of new histologic forms. Am J Surg Pathol 1999; 23: 1441–1454

Vogl HJ et al. Superparamagnetic iron oxide-enhanced versus gadolinium-enhanced MR imaging for differential diagnosis of focal liver lesions. Radiology 1996; 198: 881–887

Liver

Definition

Primary benign hormone-induced liver neoplasm.

▸ **Epidemiology**

Usually occurs in women between the ages of 20 and 40 years • Rare in men • Occurs almost exclusively in women with a long history of oral contraceptive use; there is a correlation between the duration of use and the risk of developing adenoma • Less often secondary to anabolic steroid misuse and glycogen storage disease.

▸ **Etiology, pathophysiology, pathogenesis**

Consists almost entirely of uniformly shaped liver cells arranged in strands surrounding sinusoids • Does not include bile ducts or portal venous branches • Contains Kupffer cells • *Special form:* Adenomatosis of the liver with multiple adenomas (histologically and radiologically identical).

Imaging Signs

▸ **Modality of choice**

MRI • CT (in acute hemorrhage).

▸ **Pathognomonic findings**

Smoothly marginated, hypervascular tumor • Average size is 5–10 cm • Lesions are often encapsulated and have increased fat content • Calcifications are rare, occurring in 7% of cases • Lesions larger than 5 cm tend to develop hemorrhages and necrosis (25–40% of cases).

▸ **CT findings**

Often undetectable on unenhanced scans when no hemorrhage has occurred • Marked homogeneous enhancement occurs in areas without hemorrhage, necrosis, or fatty degeneration • Acute hemorrhage appears hyperdense on the unenhanced scan and is often accompanied by perihepatic fluid.

▸ **MRI findings**

Hyperintense on unenhanced T1-weighted and T2-weighted images due to the increased fat content (in up to 75% of cases) • Marked, homogeneous enhancement in the areas without necrosis or hemorrhage • Rapid passage of contrast occurs in the portal venous and equilibrium phase • Administration of a hepatocyte-specific contrast agent in the late phase produces no enhancement • After SPIO administration, signal is decreased on T2-weighted images as lesions contain varying amounts of reticuloendothelial tissue.

▸ **Ultrasound findings**

Isoechoic or hyperechoic • Marked enhancement only in the arterial phase after contrast administration.

Clinical Aspects

▸ **Typical presentation**

Large tumors can produce a sensation of pressure • Often detected because of hemorrhage.

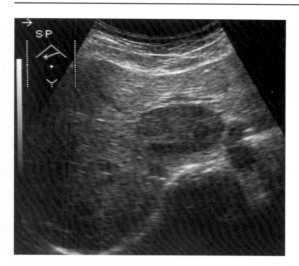

Fig. 1.19 Hepatic adenoma. Ultrasound. Inhomogeneous hypoechoic hepatic tumor immediately adjacent to the vena cava.

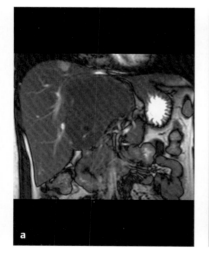

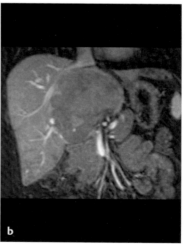

Fig. 1.20 a, b Hepatic adenoma. MR image. Lesion is slightly hypointense to surrounding liver tissue on the T2-weighted image. Hepatic veins and portal venous system are displaced. Incidental findings include a hemangioma on the dome of the liver (**a**). After contrast administration, the lesion shows slightly inhomogeneous enhancement, less than in normal liver tissue (**b**).

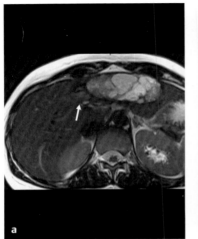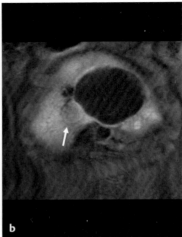

a b

Fig. 1.21 a, b Hepatic adenoma with hemorrhage. **a** T2-weighted MR image. Inhomogeneous pattern after hemorrhage in a hepatic adenoma. At the margin of the hemorrhage, a solid tumor nodule can be differentiated (arrow). **b** After contrast administration, the adenoma (arrow) is slightly better differentiated from the surrounding liver tissue. Adjacent to the lesion is a large signal void representing the hemorrhage.

▶ **Therapeutic options**
Surgical removal • Small adenomas (less than 4 cm) may be treated by percutaneous radiofrequency ablation • Discontinue oral contraceptives.

▶ **Course and prognosis**
Issue of malignant degeneration is controversial • Risk of hemorrhage is increased in larger tumors (> 5 cm) with relatively high mortality (9–21%).

▶ **What does the clinician want to know?**
Rule out focal nodular hyperplasia and HCC.

Differential Diagnosis

Focal nodular hyperplasia	– More pronounced and nodular contrast enhancement – Central enhancing "scar" – Uptake of hepatobiliary gadolinium compounds in the late phase
Hemangioma	– Iris-like contrast filling – High signal intensity on T2-weighted images
Cholangiocarcinoma	– Indentation of the liver capsule is fairly typical – Often there is late enhancement – Segmental bile ducts usually dilated
HCC	– Usually in a cirrhotic liver – Hypervascular lesion with rapid washout – AFP is raised
Hypervascular metastases	– Usually multiple, smaller focal lesions

Tips and Pitfalls

Can be misinterpreted as focal nodular hyperplasia or HCC.

Selected Literature

Dietrich CF et al. Differentiation of focal nodular hyperplasia and hepatocellular adenoma by contrast-enhanced ultrasound. Br J Radiol 2005; 78: 704–707

Grazioli L et al. Accurate differentiation of focal nodular hyperplasia from hepatic adenoma at gadobenate dimeglumine-enhanced MR imaging: prospective study. Radiology 2005; 236: 166–177

Ichikawa T et al. Hepatocellular adenoma: multiphasic CT and histopathologic findings in 25 patients. Radiology 2000; 214: 861–868

Liver

Definition
....

▶ **Epidemiology**
Most common primary tumor of the liver • Frequency is increasing • Increased incidence in southeast Asia and Africa • Primarily occurs in older people (ages 50–70 years) • Four times as common in men than in women.

▶ **Etiology, pathophysiology, pathogenesis**
Occurs in the setting of cirrhosis or chronic hepatitis B or C • Usually develops from regenerating nodules and dysplastic nodules • Accompanied by simultaneous decrease in portal venous perfusion and increase in arterial perfusion • Three forms of growth—solitary, nodular, or multifocal and/or diffuse • Important characteristics of the primary tumor include its size, number and location of foci, vascular infiltration, and spread into the bile ducts • Metastasizes to regional lymph nodes, lungs, and bone.

Imaging Signs
....

▶ **Modality of choice**
Dynamic MRI (with hepatobiliary contrast agents) • Multiphasic CT • Screening is with ultrasound and AFP monitoring.

▶ **Pathognomonic findings**
Solitary tumors, often with a capsule • Necrosis is usually present in large tumors • Diffuse tumors are often difficult to differentiate in cirrhosis • Vascular infiltration • Lymph node involvement is common (50–70% of cases) • Usually there is marked enhancement in the arterial phase (especially in undifferentiated tumors) • Rapid passage of contrast agent • Some tumors are only detectable in the late phase • Enlarged lymph nodes • Lung and bone metastases.

▶ **MRI findings**
Homogeneously hypointense on T1-weighted images, occasionally hyperintense as well due to fat, copper, and blood • Often hyperintense on T2-weighted images (intensity on T2-weighted images may increase in undifferentiated tumors) • On dynamic MRI, there is marked enhancement in the arterial phase and rapid passage of contrast agent • Gadolinium in combination with SPIO increases image precision • Hepatobiliary contrast agents can be taken up by highly differentiated tumors.

▶ **CT findings**
Slightly hypodense to surrounding liver tissue on unenhanced scans • Multiphase CT (arterial phase 20–30 seconds, parenchymal phase 40–55 seconds, and portal venous phase 70–80 seconds) shows rapid enhancement in the early arterial phase and rapid passage of contrast agent.

▶ **Ultrasound findings**
Small (< 3 cm) and differentiated tumors are usually hypoechoic • Often the echo pattern is heterogeneous • Use of contrast yields precision comparable to MRI and CT • Well suited for guiding diagnostic aspiration.

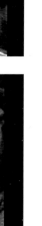

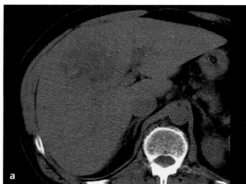

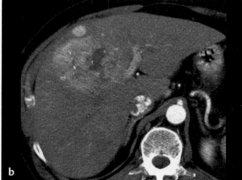

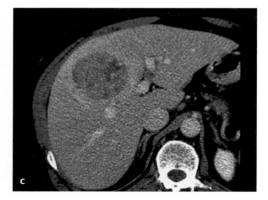

Fig. 1.22 a–c Hepatocellular carcinoma. **a** Unenhanced MR image. The tumor appears as an ill-defined hypodense lesion. **b** Early arterial phase. Small, grossly hypervascular satellite nodule. The large nodule exhibits necrotic changes that do not enhance. **c** The small satellite nodule is no longer visualized in the portal venous phase due to rapid passage of the contrast agent. The larger degenerative nodule appears hypodense.

Fig. 1.23 a–c Diffuse HCC invading the portal vein. **a** T2-weighted MR image. Hyperintense confluent nodules in the right lobe of the liver. **b** Early arterial phase. Partially enhancing nodules. **c** Portal venous phase. Nodules are now primarily hypointense. Necrotic degeneration is visualized as a central area of hypointensity.

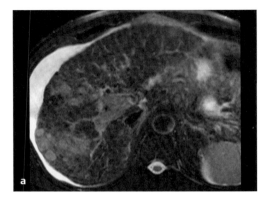

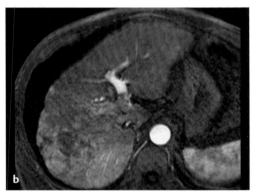

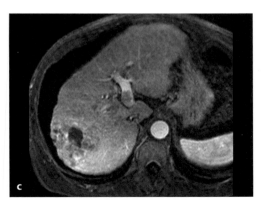

► **Angiography and nuclear medicine**
  No longer used for diagnostic imaging.
► **PET findings**
  Usually negative in HCC.

Clinical Aspects

► **Typical presentation**
  Can remain clinically asymptomatic for a long time in the setting of cirrhosis or chronic hepatitis ● Hepatomegaly with palpable mass and splenomegaly ● Abdominal pain (60–95% of cases) ● Weight loss (35–70%) ● Anorexia (25%) ● Raised AFP (sensitivity 70–80%, specificity 90%).
► **Therapeutic options**
  This depends on the size and location of the tumor and the severity of the underlying disorder ● Where surgery is possible (only 20% of cases), treatment involves resection or transplantation ● Transarterial embolization or chemoembolization ● Radiofrequency ablation (also in combined therapy).
► **Course and prognosis**
  Survival time without treatment is usually less than 1 year ● Early diagnosis and aggressive therapy improve the prognosis ● 5-year survival rate after transplantation is 60–75%, after resection 40–50%, after radiofrequency ablation about 50%, and after transarterial chemoembolization 5–20%.
► **What does the clinician want to know?**
  Early tumor diagnosis ● Staging ● Rule out pseudotumors.

Differential Diagnosis

Focal nodular hyperplasia	– More pronounced nodular contrast enhancement
	– Central enhancing "scar"
	– Uptake of hepatobiliary contrast agent in the late phase
Adenoma	– Occurs in healthy liver after years of hormone use
	– Hemorrhages are common
Hemangioma	– Iris-like pattern of enhancement
	– High signal intensity on T2-weighted images
Cholangiocarcinoma	– Indentation of the liver capsule is fairly typical
	– Contrast enhancement is usually late (10 minutes)
	– Calcifications in 20% of all cases
	– Usually associated with segmental bile duct dilation
Hypervascular metastases	– Usually multiple, smaller focal lesions

Tips and Pitfalls
....

The percentage of false negative findings is relatively high as tumors are difficult to identify in distorted liver architecture. False positive findings are also common due to regenerating nodules, arterioportal shunts, and atypical hemangiomas.

Selected Literature

Bhartia B et al. HCC in cirrhotic livers: double-contrast thin section MRI with pathologic correlation of explanted tissue. AJR 2003; 180: 577–584

Iannaccone R et al. Hepatocellular carcinoma: role of unenhanced and delayed phase multi-detector row helical CT in patients with cirrhosis. Radiology 2005; 234: 460–467

Szklaruk J et al. Imaging in the diagnosis, staging, treatment, and surveillance of hepatocellular carcinoma. AJR 2003; 180: 441–454

Valls C et al. Pretransplantation diagnosis and staging of hepatocellular carcinoma in patients with cirrhosis: value of dual-phase helical CT. AJR 2004; 182: 1011–1017

Definition

Special form of HCC that develops in a healthy liver ● Nodular internal structure with prominent strands of fibrous tissue, often (in up to 60% of cases) occurring in a stellate configuration as in focal nodular hyperplasia ● Often well differentiated ● With satellite nodules in 10–20% of cases.

▶ **Epidemiology**
Rare primary malignancy of the liver ● Accounts for 1–9% of all HCCs (up to 35% of HCCs in individuals under 50 years, without an underlying liver disorder) ● Average patient age is 20–30 years ● No sex predilection.

▶ **Etiology, pathophysiology, pathogenesis**
Occurs without an underlying liver disorder ● There are no known specific risk factors.

Imaging Signs

▶ **Modality of choice**
Dynamic MRI, multiphasic CT.

▶ **Pathognomonic findings**
Large, well-demarcated hypervascular tumor (5–20 cm) ● Exhibits broad avascular fibrotic bands that can form a stellate scar ● Necrotic areas and calcifications are often present (35–55% of cases) ● No capsule ● Tumors usually occur as solitary lesions ● Satellite nodules occur in 10–15% of cases ● Vascular infiltration is rare ● Lymph node involvement is common (50–70%).

▶ **MRI findings**
Homogeneously hypointense on T1-weighted images, heterogeneous and hyperintense on T2-weighted images ● The strands of fibrous tissue (scars) appear hypointense on all sequences ● Inhomogeneous contrast enhancement in the arterial and portal venous phases ● The scar does not enhance and is best visualized in the later phases ● SPIO is not taken up by the reticuloendothelial system.

▶ **CT findings**
Slightly hypodense to surrounding liver tissue on unenhanced scans ● Calcifications are well visualized ● Marked but inhomogeneous enhancement occurs in the arterial and portal venous phases ● The fibrotic components (and scars) do not enhance.

▶ **Ultrasound findings**
Highly heterogeneous echo pattern ● Calcifications are readily detectable ● Scar is hyperechoic.

▶ **Angiography and nuclear medicine**
No longer used.

Clinical Aspects

▶ **Typical presentation**
Large tumors can produce a sensation of pressure and pain in the upper abdomen ● Hepatomegaly with a palpable mass ● Weight loss ● Jaundice is rare, oc-

Liver

Fig. 1.24 a, b
Fibrolamellar HCC.
a CT. Inhomogene-
ous tumor of the
left hepatic lobe
that enhances
slightly more than
the normal right
lobe. Calcification
(thick arrow) and
scarring (small ar-
rows) in the tumor.
b T2-weighted MR
image. The large
liver tumor exhibits
a hyperintense
pseudocapsule and
a significantly inho-
mogeneous struc-
ture with hypoin-
tense scarring.

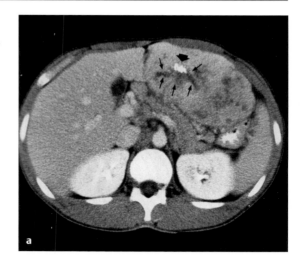

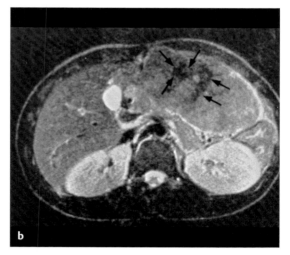

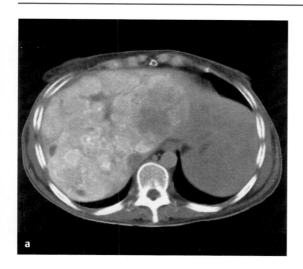

Fig. 1.25 a, b
Fibrolamellar HCC.
a CT. Large tumor
of the right hepatic
lobe showing par-
tially nodular pat-
tern of enhance-
ment.
b Unenhanced
T1-weighted MR
image. Inhomo-
geneous nodular
tumor.

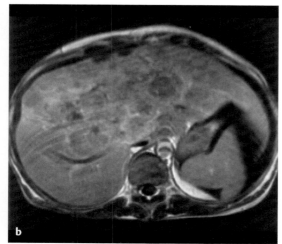

curring in 5% of cases ● AFP is rarely raised ● Transaminase levels are often slightly elevated.

▶ **Therapeutic options**

Resection or transplantation ● Adjuvant chemotherapy is indicated in advanced cases.

▶ **Course and prognosis**

Prognosis is slightly better than in the usual HCC ● The 5-year survival rate is as high as 67%.

▶ **What does the clinician want to know?**

Rule out other hypervascular tumors or changes.

Differential Diagnosis

Focal nodular hyperplasia	– More pronounced contrast enhancement – Central enhancing "scar" – Uptake of hepatobiliary gadolinium compounds in the late phase
Adenoma	– Secondary to years of hormone use – Hemorrhages are common
Hemangioma	– Iris-like contrast filling – High signal intensity on T2-weighted images
Cholangiocarcinoma	– Indentation of the liver capsule is fairly typical – Contrast enhancement is often late (10 minutes) – Segmental bile ducts are usually dilated
HCC	– Usually in a cirrhotic liver – Vascular infiltration is more common – Calcifications are rare – AFP is raised
Hypervascular metastases	– Usually multiple, smaller focal lesions

Tips and Pitfalls

May be confused with focal nodular hyperplasia ● Where biopsy is indicated, specimens should be as large as possible as there is also a risk of histologic misinterpretation as focal nodular hyperplasia or other pathology ● Biopsy should not be taken from the surface of the liver.

Selected Literature

Ichikawa T et al. Fibrolamellar hepatocellular carcinoma: Pre- and posttherapy evaluation with CT and MR imaging. Radiology 2000; 217: 145–151

McLarney JK et al. Fibrolamellar carcinoma of the liver: radiologic-pathologic correlation. RadioGraphics 1999; 19: 453–471

Soyer P et al. CT of fibrolamellar hepatocellular carcinoma. J Comput Assist Tomogr 1991; 15: 533–538

Definition

Intrahepatic tumor arising from the bile duct epithelium.

▶ **Epidemiology**
Accounts for 15% of malignant liver tumors • 20–30% of bile duct carcinomas exhibit intrahepatic growth • Rare in younger people • Usually occurs at age 50–60 years.

▶ **Etiology, pathophysiology, pathogenesis**
More common in primary sclerosing cholangitis, with intrahepatic gallstones, and, in Asia, secondary to *Clonorchis* infection • Three forms of growth—nodular exophytic, periductal infiltrative, and intraductal polypoid (rare) • Metastasizes to the lymph nodes and often infiltrates vascular structures.

Imaging Signs

▶ **Modality of choice**
Dynamic MRI, multiphasic CT.

▶ **Pathognomonic findings**
Infiltrative growth • Often there is a large intrahepatic tumor (5–15 cm in diameter) • Segmental dilation of the intrahepatic bile ducts • Occasionally spreads along the bile ducts • Retraction of the liver capsule is occasionally observed (a characteristic sign) • Calcifications occur in up to 20% of cases • Tumor enhancement occurs late and persists for a long time.

▶ **CT findings**
Hypodense on unenhanced scans • Nodular to coarse calcifications are well visualized • Arterial phase demonstrates a hypervascular halo • Enhancement is heterogeneous in the late phase, and tumor margins are often more clearly demarcated.

▶ **MRI findings**
Hypointense and inhomogeneous on T1-weighted images • Occasionally slightly hyperintense on T2-weighted images • T2-weighted images and MRCP show a narrowed lumen with peripheral dilatation • Late and variable enhancement after contrast administration • SPIO improves demarcation from liver parenchyma on T2-weighted images.

▶ **Ultrasound findings**
Heterogeneous echo pattern • Usually slightly hypoechoic to surrounding tissue (in 75% of cases) • Occasionally isoechoic or hyperechoic.

Clinical Aspects

▶ **Typical presentation**
Abdominal pain • Weight loss • Fatigue • Jaundice.

▶ **Therapeutic options**
Resection • Bile duct drainage with stent in tumors exhibiting central growth • Results are poor for transplantation.

Fig. 1.26 a, b
Cholangiocarcinoma. CT. Large, primarily avascular tumor in the early arterial (**a**) and late venous (**b**) phases.

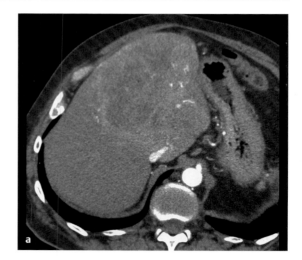

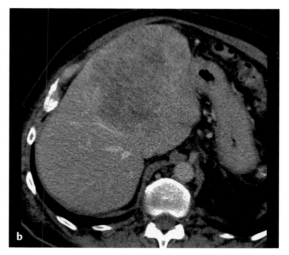

▶ **Course and prognosis**

Poor prognosis • Less than 20% of tumors are resectable.

▶ **What does the clinician want to know?**

Rule out HCC • Is tumor resectable?

Differential Diagnosis

Fibrolamellar HCC	– Usually a large tumor with necrotic areas and calcifications
	– Contains scars that have low signal intensity on T2-weighted images and do not enhance
HCC	– Usually in a cirrhotic liver
	– Vascular infiltration is more common
	– AFP is raised
Metastases	– Usually no cholestasis
	– Usually no late contrast enhancement
Alveolar echinococcosis	– Often associated with small or large cysts

Tips and Pitfalls

Failing to obtain late images after contrast administration (5–10 minutes).

Selected Literature

Lim JH et al. Cholangiocarcinoma: morphologic classification according to growth pattern and imaging findings. AJR 2003; 181: 819–927

Loyer EM et al. Hepatocellular carcinoma and intrahepatic peripheral cholangiocarcinoma: enhancemant patterns with quadruple phase helical CT—a comparative study. Radiology 1999; 212: 866–875

Soyer P. Imaging of intrahepatic cholangiocarcinoma: Peripheral cholangiocarcinoma. AJR 1995; 165: 1427–1431

Definition

▶ **Epidemiology**
Most common malignancy of the liver (20 times more common than primary liver tumors).

▶ **Etiology, pathophysiology, pathogenesis**
Seeding occurs via the systemic or portal circulatory system • Most common primary tumors are lung, breast, gastrointestinal tract, pancreas, melanoma, and sarcoma.

Imaging Signs

▶ **Modality of choice**
Ultrasound, CT, MRI.

▶ **Pathognomonic findings**
Isolated or multiple focal lesions • Hypovascular or hypervascular (usually like the primary tumor) • Occasionally associated with metastases in lymph nodes and other organs • Diffuse dissemination is rare • Large numbers of metastases cause liver enlargement.

▶ **Ultrasound findings**
Usually hypoechoic focal lesions in the liver, less often hyperechoic • Occasionally there will be a hypoechoic halo • Metastases of cystic tumors may appear cystic • Ultrasound contrast studies provide high-resolution realtime images of vascularization • Ultrasound is the modality of choice for all those tumors in which CT or MRI is not performed as the initial study (such as breast carcinoma and melanoma).

▶ **CT findings**
Tumor is often nearly indistinguishable from the surrounding liver tissue on unenhanced scans • Hypovascular metastases appear hypodense after contrast administration, often with a hyperdense halo • Hypervascular metastases show marked enhancement in the arterial phase • The liver is included in staging examinations for abdominal and thoracic tumors.

▶ **MRI findings**
Hypointense or isointense on T1-weighted images • Moderate to intense signal on T2-weighted images • Metastases of neuroendocrine tumors can appear extremely hyperintense on T2-weighted images, mimicking cysts or hemangiomas • Hypovascular metastases often have a hypointense center and a slightly hyperintense halo • Hypervascular metastases show marked enhancement in the arterial phase • After administration of hepatobiliary contrast agents, only healthy liver tissue enhances in the late phase • After administration of SPIO, only healthy liver tissue enhances as metastases do not have a reticuloendothelial system.

▶ **PET, PET-CT findings**
Usually there is increased uptake of FDG • However, diagnostic precision is limited with metastases smaller than 1 cm.

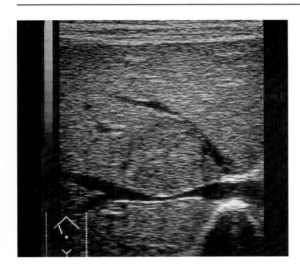

Fig. 1.27 Liver metastases. Ultrasound scan. Slightly hypoechoic metastasis of a bronchial carcinoma. Compression of hepatic veins.

Clinical Aspects

▶ **Typical presentation**
Symptoms are unspecific ● Weight loss ● Fatigue ● Jaundice ● Transaminase, bilirubin, alkaline phosphatase, and LDH levels are slightly raised.

▶ **Therapeutic options**
Solitary focal lesions are resected (possible in 5% of cases) or treated with radiofrequency ablation ● Transarterial chemoembolization is also an option with metastases of neuroendocrine tumors ● Diffuse involvement is treated with systemic chemotherapy.

▶ **Course and prognosis**
Prognosis is poor ● Depends on the underlying disease.

▶ **What does the clinician want to know?**
Number, location, and size of the metastases.

Differential Diagnosis

Hemangioma of the liver	– Iris-like pattern of enhancement
	– Markedly hyperintense on T2-weighted images
Hepatic cysts	– Do not enhance
	– Markedly hyperintense on T2-weighted images
Liver abscesses	– Usually exhibit a broad halo
	– Fever

Fig. 1.28 a–c Small metastasis of the right hepatic lobe.
a CT. Central enhancement after contrast administration.
b MR image. Homogeneous enhancement.
c T2-weighted image after administration of SPIO. The metastasis appears hyperintense.

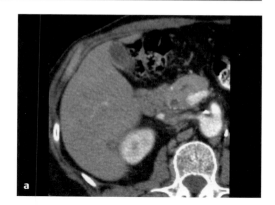

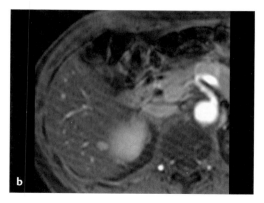

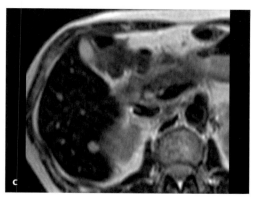

Liver

Tips and Pitfalls
. . . .

Small liver lesions on CT are too often interpreted as metastases even in patients with malignant disease (50% of focal lesions less than 1.5 cm are benign) • Imaging hypervascular metastases in an unsuitable phase is a common error.

Selected Literature

Jones EC et al. The frequency and significance of small (less than or equal to 15 mm) hepatic lesions detected by CT. AJR 1992; 158: 535–539

Larsen RE et al. Hypervascular malignant liver lesions: comparison of various MR imaging pulse sequences and dynamic CT. Radiology 1994; 192: 393–399

Ward J et al. Liver metastases in candidates for hepatic resection: comparison of helical CT and Gadolinium- and SPIO-enhanced MRI. Radiology 2005; 237: 170–180

Definition

▶ **Epidemiology**
Primary lymphomas of the liver are rare • They account for 0.4–1% of all extra-nodal lymphomas • Average age is 50–60 years • More common in men • However, the liver is the most commonly affected organ in malignant lympho-mas (5–10% of cases in Hodgkin disease, 15–40% in non-Hodgkin lymphomas).

▶ **Etiology, pathophysiology, pathogenesis**
More commonly occurs secondary to transplantation and in AIDS patients.

Imaging Signs

▶ **Modality of choice**
MRI, CT.

▶ **Pathognomonic findings**
– *Primary lymphoma:* Well-demarcated tumors • Usually solitary • Large tu-mors with central necrosis or fibrosis • Rarely there is diffuse dissemination.
– *Secondary lymphoma:* Enlarged liver • Diffuse infiltrative growth or multiple nodules • Known Hodgkin or non-Hodgkin lymphoma.

▶ **MRI findings**
Hypointense or isointense on T1-weighted images, hyperintense on T2-weighted images • Slight enhancement after intravenous gadolinium injection • SPIO is not taken up.

▶ **CT findings**
Slightly hypodense to surrounding liver tissue on unenhanced scans • Hypovas-cular or hypervascular tumors are visualized after contrast administration • Central areas of fibrosis and necrosis enhance slightly with contrast • Diffuse in-volvement appears as generalized reduced enhancement, as in fatty infiltration of the liver.

▶ **Ultrasound findings**
Usually there is a hypoechoic to anechoic mass.

▶ **PET findings**
Marked FDG uptake.

Clinical Aspects

▶ **Typical presentation**
Symptoms are unspecific • Pain in the upper abdomen • Hepatomegaly • Sys-temic symptoms occur in 50% of cases (fever, night sweats, and weight loss) • AFP is rarely raised • Transaminase levels are often slightly raised.

▶ **Therapeutic options**
Solitary lesions are resected • Chemotherapy and radiation therapy.

▶ **Course and prognosis**
Prognosis is poor in immunosuppressed patients • Mean survival time is 1.5 years.

▶ **What does the clinician want to know?**
Rule out other tumors or lesions.

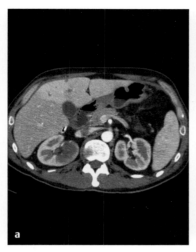 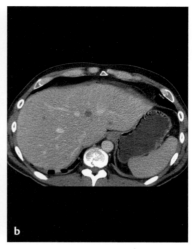

Fig. 1.29 a, b　Lymphoma of the right kidney and liver. MR image. Small hypodense focal lesions in the early arterial (**a**) and portal venous (**b**) phases.

Differential Diagnosis

Focal nodular hyperplasia	– Marked nodular contrast enhancement – Central enhancing "scar" – Uptake of hepatobiliary gadolinium compounds in the late phase
Adenoma	– Grossly hypervascular tumor – Secondary to years of hormone use
HCC	– Usually in a cirrhotic liver – Hypervascular lesion with rapid washout – AFP is raised
Metastases	– Usually there is a known primary disorder
Fatty infiltration of the liver	– Reduced signal intensity on T1-weighted images (out-of-phase GE sequence)

Tips and Pitfalls

Can be confused with HCC ● Biopsy can also be misinterpreted as a poorly differentiated carcinoma.

Selected Literature

Fukuya T et al. MRI of primary lymphoma of the liver. J Comput Assist Tomogr 1993; 17: 596–598

Fig. 1.30 a, b Lymphoma of the liver. Large hypodense lymphoma of the liver exhibiting a bizarre pattern of enhancement in the center after contrast administration.

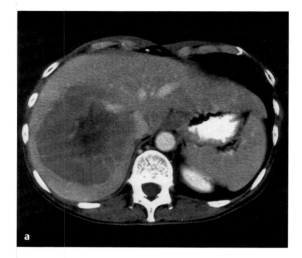

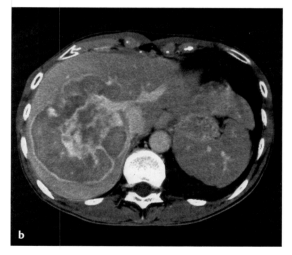

Gazelle GS et al. US, CT, and MRI of primary and secondary liver lymphoma. J Comput Assist Tomogr 1994; 18: 412–415

Kelekis NL et al. Focal hepatic lymphoma: magnetic resonance demonstration using current techniques including gadolinium enhancement. Magn Reson Imaging 1997; 15: 625–636

Definition

Venous thrombosis with hepatic congestion.

▶ **Epidemiology**
Rare disorder • Occurs in all age groups • Slightly more common in females than in men.

▶ **Etiology, pathophysiology, pathogenesis**
Often idiopathic • Known causes include coagulation disorders, pregnancy, oral contraceptives, infections, and tumor thrombosis • Occlusion at the level of the inferior vena cava or in the large intrahepatic or centrilobular veins (venous occlusive disease) • Complete, segmental, or subsegmental occlusion • Occlusion leads to increased sinusoidal pressure with slowing or reversal of portal venous blood flow.

Imaging Signs

▶ **Modality of choice**
Ultrasound, MRI, CT.

▶ **Pathognomonic findings**
Ascites • Hypertrophy of the caudate lobe (which has its own venous drainage system) • Increasing atrophy of the peripheral portions of the liver • Regenerating nodules and dysplastic nodules • Collaterals.

▶ **MRI findings**
Acute stage: Periphery of the liver appears hypointense on T1-weighted images and hyperintense on T2-weighted images (edema) • Slight enhancement in the peripheral areas • Ascites.
Subacute stage: Increased, highly heterogeneous enhancement in the peripheral areas of the liver.
Chronic stage: Hypointense on T1-weighted and T2-weighted images in the peripheral areas of the liver (fibrosis) • The marked differences in contrast enhancement between the peripheral and central areas of the liver gradually even out • Massive hypertrophy of the caudate lobe • Prominent collaterals • Regenerating nodules and dysplastic nodules show high signal intensity on T1-weighted images and moderate to low intensity on T2-weighted images • Nodules enhance during the arterial phase.

▶ **CT findings**
Acute stage: Diffusely enlarged liver with reduced radiodensity • Narrowing of the vena cava or intrahepatic veins with hyperdense contents (acute thrombus) • Inhomogeneous mottled parenchyma after contrast administration • Caudate lobe shows pronounced enhancement • Reduced enhancement in the peripheral areas of the liver.
Subacute stage: Increasingly marked enhancement of the peripheral areas of the liver.
Chronic stage: Increasing hypertrophy of the caudate lobe and atrophy of the peripheral areas of the liver • Large regenerating nodules develop, which enhance during the arterial phase • Collaterals.

Liver

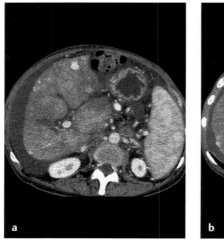 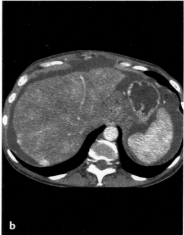

Fig. 1.31 a, b   Budd–Chiari syndrome. CT. The parenchyma appears inhomogeneously mottled in the arterial and venous phases and its overall density is reduced. Isolated degenerative and/or dysplastic nodules showing marked enhancement. Hypertrophic caudate lobe and ascites.

▶ **Ultrasound findings**
Color Doppler shows narrowing of the hepatic veins without blood flow ● "Two-color" liver veins with intrahepatic collaterals ● Slow hepatofugal blood flow in the portal vein ● Resistance index (RI) of the hepatic artery is higher than 0.75.
▶ **Venographic findings**
Occluded hepatic veins ● No longer used for diagnostic imaging.

Clinical Aspects

▶ **Typical presentation**
Severe pain in the upper abdomen ● Vomiting ● Hepatomegaly ● Ascites ● Slight jaundice ● Clinical course is often insidious.
▶ **Therapeutic options**
Management of the coagulation disorder ● TIPS ● Extreme cases may require liver transplantation.
▶ **Course and prognosis**
Depend on the severity of the venous occlusion ● Total thrombotic occlusion can cause liver failure ● Portal hypertension can lead to hemorrhage from esophageal varices.
▶ **What does the clinician want to know?**
Cause and severity of the disorder.

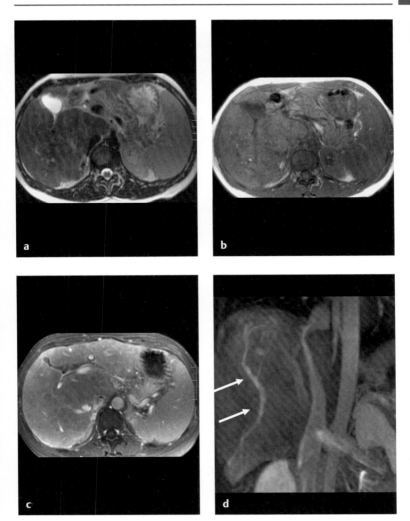

Fig. 1.32 a–d Budd–Chiari syndrome. Unenhanced T2-weighted MR image (**a**). Inhomogeneous picture with strands of scarring and marked hypertrophy of the caudate lobe. Unenhanced T1-weighted MR image (**b**). Findings are identical to T2-weighted sequence. After contrast administration (**c**). Small hypointense nodules and hypertrophy of the caudate lobe are more clearly visualized. Visualization of vascular structures (**d**). Constriction of the vena cava at the venous confluence. Normal hepatic veins are not detectable; collateral veins (arrows) are visualized instead.

Differential Diagnosis

Cirrhosis of the liver	– Known etiology (alcoholism, hepatitis, cholangitis)
	– Chronic disorder
	– Blood flow in hepatic veins
	– Splenomegaly

Tips and Pitfalls

Misjudging the severity of the disorder.

Selected Literature

Brancatelli G et al. Benign regenerative nodules in Budd–Chiari syndrome and other vascular disorders of the liver. Radiologic-pathologic and clinical correlation. RadioGraphics 2002; 22: 847–862

Kane R et al. Diagnosis of Budd–Chiari syndrome: comparison between sonography and MR angiography. Radiology 1995; 195: 117–121

Noone TC et al. Budd–Chiari syndrome: spectrum of appearances of acute, subacute, and chronic disease with magnetic resonance imaging. J Magn Reson Imaging 2000; 11: 44–50

Definition

▶ **Epidemiology**
Rare but life-threatening acute situation.
▶ **Etiology, pathophysiology, pathogenesis**
Traumatic etiology with or without underlying liver disease • Spontaneous hemorrhages can occur in tumors (hepatic adenoma, HCC, giant hemangioma), vascular disorders (Osler–Weber–Rendu disease, idiopathic aneurysm, periarteritis nodosa), coagulation disorders, and HELLP syndrome in the setting of preeclampsia.

Imaging Signs

▶ **Modality of choice**
CT, ultrasound.
▶ **Pathognomonic findings**
Increase in liver size • Fluid accumulation in the hepatic parenchyma, the subcapsular region, and often in the perihepatic region • Leakage of contrast medium into parenchyma • Tears in the parenchyma (after trauma).
▶ **CT findings**
Acute hemorrhage is hyperdense, chronic hemorrhage hypodense • Traumatic lacerations are readily detectable, especially after contrast administration • Findings in acute hemorrhage include extravasated contrast medium • In a ruptured tumor, the underlying focal lesions are usually no longer detectable.
▶ **MRI findings**
Examination takes too long to be of use in severe acute hemorrhage • Minor hemorrhages may be incidental findings in patients with abdominal pain • Signal intensity depends on the age of the hemorrhage • T1-weighted images of acute hemorrhage show areas of high signal intensity.
▶ **Ultrasound findings**
Fresh blood is anechoic, becomes hyperechoic after 24 hours, and hypoechoic after 4–5 days • After several weeks, septa can be detected.
▶ **Angiographic findings**
Demonstrates extravasation of blood • Therapeutic angiography may be indicated.

Clinical Aspects

▶ **Typical presentation**
Acute pain • Symptoms of acute blood loss including hypovolemic shock.
▶ **Therapeutic options**
Transarterial embolization • Surgical repair.
▶ **Course and prognosis**
This depends on the underlying disorder and the severity of the acute hemorrhage • Hemorrhages extending into the abdominal cavity are associated with increased mortality.

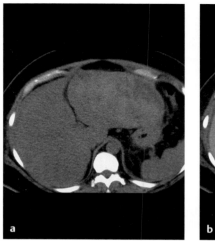 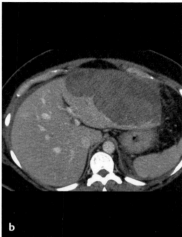

Fig. 1.33 a, b   Extensive hemorrhage in the parenchyma of the left hepatic lobe. **a** Unenhanced CT. The hemorrhage is identifiable by slightly hyperdense areas. **b** After contrast administration the hematoma is clearly differentiated from the surrounding liver tissue. The cause of the bleeding cannot be identified on the images.

▶ **What does the clinician want to know?**
Extent of the hemorrhage ● Rupture of the liver with bleeding into the abdominal cavity ● Are interventional treatments possible?

Differential Diagnosis

HCC	– Usually in a cirrhotic liver
	– AFP is raised
Hepatocellular adenoma	– In younger women with a history of many years of oral contraceptive use
HELLP syndrome	– Variant of preeclampsia
Vascular disease	– An aneurysm is occasionally demonstrated
	– Large-caliber arteries
Coagulation disorder	– Low thrombocyte count
	– Coagulation defects
	– Recurrent episodes of bleeding

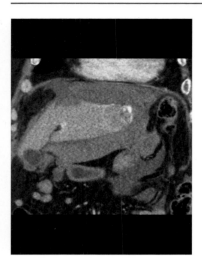

Fig. 1.34 CT. Spontaneous perihepatic bleeding from an HCC nodule.

Tips and Pitfalls

Misinterpretation of intraabdominal bleeding as ascites.

Selected Literature

Casillas VJ et al. Imaging of nontraumatic hemorrhagic hepatic lesions. RadioGraphics 2000; 20: 367–388

Flowers BF et al. Ruptured hepatic adenoma: a spectrum of presentation and treatment. Am Surg 1990; 56: 380–384

Pretorius ES et al. CT of hemorrhagic complications of anticoagulant therapy. J Comput Assist Tomogr 1997; 21: 44–51

Definition

▶ **Epidemiology**
Rare developmental anomaly • In one autopsy series, the incidence was about 1:4000.

▶ **Etiology, pathophysiology, pathogenesis**
Congenital malformation • Two forms exist:
  – The primordium of the cystic duct divides, forming a septated gallbladder or a Y-shaped double gallbladder.
  – Double primordia lead to an accessory gallbladder with its own cystic duct, which drains either into the common bile duct (ductal type, 50% of cases) or, less often, into the right or left hepatic duct (trabecular type, less than 5% of cases).

Imaging Signs

▶ **Modality of choice**
Ultrasound, MRCP.

▶ **Pathognomonic findings**
Two gallbladders, usually parallel to each other • The second gallbladder can lie entirely within the liver.

▶ **Ultrasound findings**
Two gallbladder lumina • The orifice of the cystic duct is usually not visualized.

▶ **MRCP findings**
Two gallbladder lumina, with better visualization of the cystic duct • Clearly shows communication with the biliary system on T1-weighted images after administration of hepatobiliary contrast agents.

▶ **ERCP or PTC findings**
Clearly shows the anomaly • Invasive procedure that is no longer indicated.

Clinical Aspects

▶ **Typical presentation**
Persistence of biliary symptoms after cholecystectomy • Incidental finding on CT or MRI.

▶ **Therapeutic options**
Cholecystectomy.

▶ **Course and prognosis**
Benign disorder.

▶ **What does the clinician want to know?**
Gallstones • Preoperative evidence of two gallbladders and the type of anomaly.

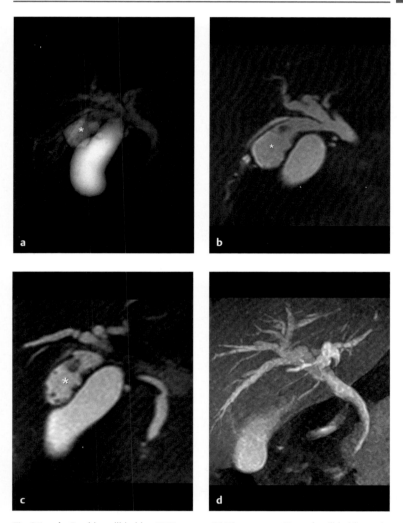

Fig. 2.1 a–d Double gallbladder. MR image, **a** RARE sequence. Normal gallbladder and second gallbladder (*) communicating with the normal right hepatic duct (**b, c**). On MIP images (HASTE) two adjacent slices show the origin of the second gallbladder from the right hepatic duct and the concretions in the second gallbladder. **d** After administration of manganese DPDP, only the normal gallbladder and extrahepatic and intrahepatic bile ducts fill with contrast.

Differential Diagnosis

Hepatic cysts	– Round shape
	– Do not communicate with the biliary system
Choledochal cyst (type II)	– Usually indistinguishable

Tips and Pitfalls

Can be misdiagnosed as a cyst, especially after cholecystectomy.

Selected Literature

Goiney RC et al. Sonography of gallbladder duplication and differential considerations. AJR 1985; 145: 241–243

Hishinuma M et al. Double gallbladder. J Gastroenterol Hepatol 2004; 19: 233–235

Milot L et al. Double gallbladder diagnosed on contrast-enhanced MR cholangiography with mangafodipirtrisodium. AJR 2005; 184: S88–S90

Definition

▶ **Epidemiology**
Gallstones occur in 10–15% of the population ● Bile duct stones are found in 10% of patients with symptomatic gallstones ● *Risk factors:* Overweight ("fat"), female sex ("female"), multiple pregnancies ("fertile"), age over 40 ("forty"), genetic disposition ("fair"), diabetes mellitus, bile acid malabsorption (as in Crohn disease).

▶ **Etiology, pathophysiology, pathogenesis**
Increased cholesterol concentration and/or decreased concentrations of bile acids and phospholipids lead to formation of microcrystals ● Decreased motility and inflammation are conducive to stone formation ● Size range is 1–20 mm ● Cholesterol stones mixed with bilirubin and calcium salts account for 80% of all stones ● 10% are pure cholesterol stones ● 10% are pigment stones ● Bile duct stones usually originate in the gallbladder ● Only brown pigment stones arise directly in the bile ducts (in strictures and ductal anomalies).

Imaging Signs

▶ **Modality of choice**
Ultrasound ● CT (with complications) ● MRCP (in bile duct stones).

▶ **Pathognomonic findings**
  – *Gallbladder stones:* Intraluminal spherical formations along the walls ● Mobile.
  – *Bile duct stones:* Intraluminal spherical formations ● With or without obstruction.
  – *Complications of cholelithiasis:* Hydrops of the gallbladder ● Acute cholecystitis and cholangitis ● Gallbladder perforation ● Obstructive jaundice ● Acute pancreatitis.

▶ **Ultrasound findings**
Bright echodense reflections, usually with a posterior acoustic shadow ● Bile duct stones are more difficult to demonstrate and in 10% of all cases show no posterior acoustic shadow ● Diagnostic precision is higher in dilated bile ducts.

▶ **MRI findings**
Filling defects with low signal intensity in the gallbladder and bile ducts on T2-weighted images and on MRCP ● Not suitable for small stones (< 3 mm) ● Impingement of stones can make it difficult to properly characterize an obstruction ● In certain cases, the bile ducts are better visualized on T1-weighted images after administration of manganese or hepatobiliary contrast agents.

▶ **CT findings**
Density of the gallstones is highly variable (ranging from the density of fatty tissue, to that of soft tissue and of calcification) ● 75–85% of all stones contain enough calcium oxide to distinguish them from bile ● Thin-slice CT and reconstruction along the bile ducts (multidetector CT) facilitate diagnosis of bile duct stones ● Impinging gallstones lead to bile duct obstruction and ring enhancement in the bile duct wall after intravenous contrast injection ● In certain cases,

Fig. 2.2 Cholecys-
tolithiasis. Ultra-
sound. Small con-
cretion in the infun-
dibulum of the gall-
bladder without a
shadow (migrates
into the fundus of
the gallbladder
when the patient
assumes a sitting
position).

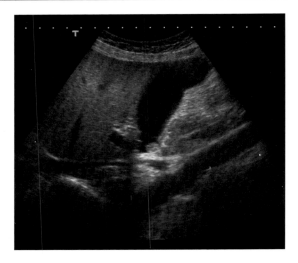

administration of hepatobiliary contrast agents is indicated to identify stones
without calcification (CT cholangiography).

▶ **ERCP findings**
Filling defects in the bile ducts • Therapeutic ERCP is indicated for symptomatic
bile duct stones.

▶ **Endosonographic findings**
Very sensitive study for demonstrating bile duct stones • However, it does not
allow extraction in the same session.

Clinical Aspects

▶ **Typical presentation**
Postprandial sensation of pressure • Dull pain in the upper abdomen, often after
consuming certain foods such as fatty foods or coffee • Biliary colic is usually attributable to transient obstruction of the cystic duct • Tenderness on palpation
of the right upper abdomen • With bile duct stones, obstruction usually leads to
cholangitis characterized by colic, jaundice, vomiting, and fever.

▶ **Therapeutic options**
Cholecystectomy is indicated for symptomatic gallbladder stones • Endoscopic
stone extraction is indicated for bile duct stones • When an endoscopic approach
is not feasible, percutaneous drainage and extraction are indicted (for example
percutaneous cholangioscopy and contact lithotripsy).

▶ **Course and prognosis**
Fifteen to 20 percent of all patients with gallbladder stones develop symptoms •
Mortality of complications is less than 1%.

Gallbladder and Biliary Tract

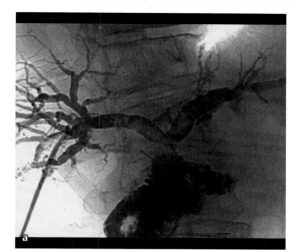

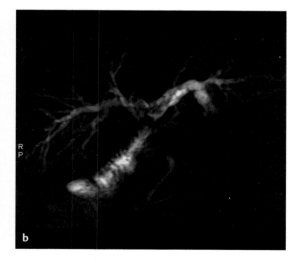

Fig. 2.3 a, b
Post-biliodigestive
anastomosis.
a PTC. Multiple
concretions in right
and left bile ducts
before the anasto-
mosis.
b MRCP. The con-
cretions are visual-
ized as signal voids.

▶ **What does the clinician want to know?**
Stones in the bile duct • Complications.

Differential Diagnosis

Tumor obstruction	– Considerably dilated bile duct
	– Depending on the type of tumor, the pancreatic duct may also be grossly dilated
	– Direct visualization of a tumor (pancreas, bile duct, or papilla of Vater)
Stenosing papillitis	– No evidence of a tumor
	– Pancreatic duct is normal or slightly dilated
	– Chronic symptoms
	– Bile duct usually tapered
Primary sclerosing cholangitis	– "Beading" of the extrahepatic and intrahepatic bile ducts
	– Fibrotic changes in the liver
Bile duct papillomas	– Multiple small intraluminal polyps
	– Slightly enhancing
	– Not mobile
Sarcoma botryoides	– In children (very rare)
	– Filling defects resembling bunches of grapes
	– No calcifications

Tips and Pitfalls

Choice of modality for demonstrating bile duct stones depends on the pretest probability (ERCP is indicated for high probability, MRCP for low probability).

Selected Literature

Aubé C et al. MR cholangiopancreatography versus endoscopic sonography in suspected common bile duct lithiasis: a prospective, comparative study. AJR 2005; 184: 55–62

Kim HC et al. Multislice CT cholangiography using thin-slab minimum intensity projection and multiplanar reformation in the evaluation of patients with suspected biliary obstruction: preliminary experience. Clin Imaging 2005; 29: 46–54

Soto JA et al. Detection of choledocholithiasis with MR cholangiography: comparison of three-dimensional fast spin-echo and single and multi-section half-Fourier rapid acquisition with relaxation enhancement sequences. Radiology 2000; 215: 737–745

Definition

Nonneoplastic, noninflammatory polypoid lesion of the gallbladder wall.

▶ **Epidemiology**
Most common polypoid pathology of the gallbladder wall • Usually multiple • More common in women • Age predilection is 40–50 years.

▶ **Etiology, pathophysiology, pathogenesis**
Polypoid form of cholesterosis as opposed to the diffuse form known as strawberry gallbladder • Composed of cholesterol-laden macrophages covered by normal epithelium • Polypoid structures can break off and become mobile like stones • Only rarely associated with gallstones.

Imaging Signs

▶ **Modality of choice**
Ultrasound.

▶ **Pathognomonic findings**
Small round polyp on the gallbladder wall • Occasionally exhibits a short pedicle • Usually measures 5–7 mm, rarely larger than 10 mm • Multiple polyps are common.

▶ **Ultrasound findings**
Usually there is a markedly hyperechoic nodule on the gallbladder wall • Usually no acoustic shadow, occasionally discrete acoustic shadow • Does not move when the patient changes position • Larger polyps are not very dense but contain markedly dense foci.

▶ **MRCP findings**
Polypoid filling defect in the lumen of the gallbladder.

▶ **CT findings**
As bile and cholesterol polyps are nearly isodense, the lesions are usually not detectable.

Clinical Aspects

▶ **Typical presentation**
Usually asymptomatic.

▶ **Therapeutic options**
No treatment.

▶ **Course and prognosis**
Invariably benign.

▶ **What does the clinician want to know?**
Exclude neoplastic polyps.

Fig. 2.4   Cholesterol polyps. Ultrasound. Hypoechoic polypoid lesions on the gallbladder wall.

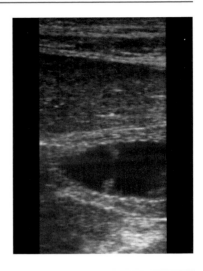

Fig. 2.5   Small hyperechoic cholesterol polyp on the anterior wall of the gallbladder.

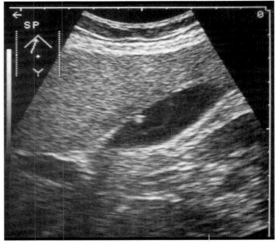

Differential Diagnosis

Gallbladder adenoma	– Usually larger than 7–8 mm – Often solitary – Surface often resembles a cauliflower
Small gallbladder stones	– Move when the patient changes position
Adenocarcinoma	– Usually much larger – Irregular thickening of the gallbladder wall

Tips and Pitfalls

Can be misdiagnosed as adenoma, leading to unnecessary cholecystectomy.

Selected Literature

Levy AD et al. Benign tumors and tumorlike lesions of the gallbladder and extrahepatic bile ducts: Radiologic-pathologic correlation. RadioGraphics 2002; 22: 387–413

Owen CC et al. Gallbladder polyps, cholesterolosis, adenomyomatosis, and acute acalculous cholecystitis. Semin Gastrointest Dis 2003; 14: 178–188

Sugyama M et al. Large cholesterol polyps of the gallbladder: diagnosis by means of US and endoscopic ultrasound. Radiology 1995; 42: 800–810

Definition

Polypoid neoplasm of the gallbladder wall.

▶ **Epidemiology**

Most common benign tumor of the gallbladder ● Usually solitary ● Familial polyposis and Peutz–Jeghers syndrome are more often associated with adenomas in the gallbladder and bile ducts ● More common in women.

▶ **Etiology, pathophysiology, pathogenesis**

Often associated with gallstones and cholecystitis (> 50% of cases) ● There seems to be an adenoma-carcinoma sequence ● The probability of malignant degeneration correlates with the size of the lesion.

Imaging Signs

▶ **Modality of choice**

Ultrasound.

▶ **Pathognomonic findings**

Pediculate or broad-based polyp arising from the gallbladder wall ● Surface is smooth or resembles a cauliflower ● Rarely larger than 2 cm ● In 10% of cases, multiple adenomas are present.

▶ **Ultrasound findings**

Polypoid mass of medium echogenicity ● No acoustic shadow ● Does not move when the patient changes position.

▶ **MRI with MRCP**

Polypoid filling defect in the lumen of the gallbladder that enhances with contrast.

▶ **CT findings**

Polypoid filling defect in the lumen of the gallbladder, isodense to soft tissue, which enhances with contrast.

▶ **ERCP**

No longer used as a primary diagnostic imaging modality.

Clinical Aspects

▶ **Typical presentation**

Usually asymptomatic.

▶ **Therapeutic options**

Cholecystectomy due to the risk of malignant degeneration (in lesions over 1 cm in diameter).

▶ **Course and prognosis**

Benign adenomas heal completely after cholecystectomy ● The prognosis of malignant polyps depends on the stage.

▶ **What does the clinician want to know?**

Rule out polypoid cholesterol deposits.

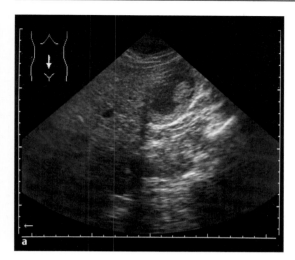

Fig. 2.6 a, b
Adenoma of the gallbladder. Ultrasound. Polypoid mass in the lumen of the gallbladder (**a**). Surgical specimen (**b**).

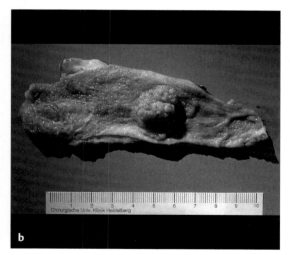

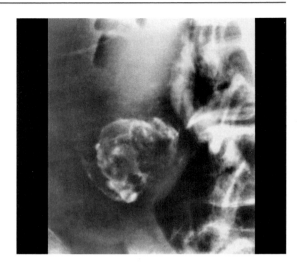

Fig. 2.7 Adenoma of the gallbladder. ERCP. Irregular filling defect in the fundus of the gallbladder caused by an adenoma measuring nearly 3 cm. Findings also include concretions in the gallbladder lumen.

Differential Diagnosis

Polypoid cholesterol deposits	– Usually not larger than 7–8 mm
	– Usually occur as multiple lesions
	– Occasionally produce a discrete acoustic shadow
Noncalcified gallbladder stones	– Move when the patient changes position
Heterotypic lesions	– Occasionally symptomatic (in gastric and pancreatic tissue)
	– Morphologically indistinguishable
Lipoma	– CT density and MRI signal intensity of fat

Tips and Pitfalls

May be misdiagnosed as polypoid cholesterol deposit.

Selected Literature

Brambs HJ et al. Großes Adenom der Gallenblase. Fortschr Röntgenstr 1986; 145: 475–477

Furukawa H et al. CT evaluation of small polypoid lesions of the gallbladder. Hepatogastroenterology 1995; 42: 800–810

Levy AD et al. Benign tumors and tumorlike lesions of the gallbladder and extrahepatic bile ducts: Radiologic-pathologic correlation. RadioGraphics 2002; 22: 387–413

Definition

Idiopathic noninflammatory and nontumorous thickening of the gallbladder wall.

▶ **Epidemiology**
Usually an incidental finding in people 40–50 years of age ● Does not occur in children ● No sex predilection ● Prevalence is 2–5%.

▶ **Etiology, pathophysiology, pathogenesis**
It is thought that increased intraluminal pressure leads to thickening of the gallbladder wall in the same way that diverticulosis of the colon leads to diverticula and thickening of the intestinal wall ● Classified as a type of hyperplastic cholecystosis ● Hyperplasia of the mucosa, thickening of the muscular layer, and diverticula (dilated Rokitansky–Aschoff sinuses) ● There are three forms—generalized (diffuse), segmental (annular), and localized (adenomyoma, usually in the fundus).

Imaging Signs

▶ **Modality of choice**
Ultrasound, MRCP.

▶ **Pathognomonic findings**
Circumscribed or generalized thickening of the wall ● Smooth outer contours ● Small cystic intramural changes ● Contractility is preserved or increased.

▶ **Ultrasound findings**
Circumscribed or generalized thickening of the wall with hypoechoic or hyperechoic inclusions ● Administration of cholecystokinin analogs produces pronounced contraction.

▶ **MRI and MRCP**
A row of diverticula in the thickened wall produces a "string of pearls" gallbladder (generalized form) ● Hourglass gallbladder with circular thickening of the wall and narrowing of the lumen (segmental form) ● Polypoid filling defect in the fundus of the gallbladder (localized form) ● After contrast administration, there is marked enhancement in the mucosa in the early arterial phase.

▶ **CT findings**
Circumscribed or generalized thickening of the wall ● Smooth outer contour ● Layers of the wall are detectable.

▶ **Oral cholecystographic and ERCP findings**
Findings identical to MRCP.

Clinical Aspects

▶ **Typical presentation**
Usually asymptomatic ● Indistinct pain in the right upper abdomen ● Occasionally persistent, colicky pain due to hypertrophy of the musculature.

▶ **Therapeutic options**
Symptomatic cases are treated by cholecystectomy.

Fig. 2.8 Adeno-myomatosis of the gallbladder. ERCP. "String of pearls" sign of contrast filling of the Rokitan-sky–Aschoff sinuses and narrowed lumen of the infundibulum of the gallbladder.

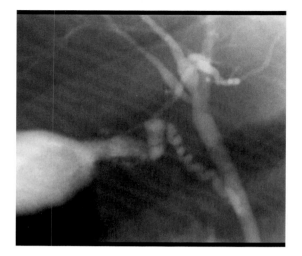

Fig. 2.9 Adeno-myoma of the fundus of the gallbladder. CT. Smooth contours (long arrow). Small gallbladder stones (short arrow).

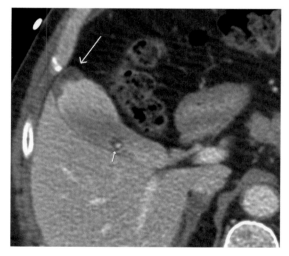

▶ **Course and prognosis**
Benign disorder.
▶ **What does the clinician want to know?**
Exclude chronic cholecystitis and gallbladder carcinoma • Contractility of the gallbladder.

Differential Diagnosis

Gallbladder carcinoma	– Irregular thickening of the gallbladder walls with irregular outer contours
	– Early infiltration of the liver
Chronic cholecystitis	– Usually typical clinical signs with gallbladder stones
	– No diverticula

Tips and Pitfalls

Can be misdiagnosed as gallbladder carcinoma.

Selected Literature

Brambs HJ et al. Sonographisches Bild der Adenomyomatose der Gallenblase. Fortschr Röntgenstr 1990; 153: 633–636
Haradome H et al. The pearl necklace sign: an imaging sign of adenomyomatosis of the gallbladder at MRCP. Radiology 2003; 227: 80–88
Yoshimitsu K et al. MR diagnosis of adenomyomatosis of the gallbladder and differentiation from gallbladder carcinoma: importance of showing Rokitansky–Aschoff sinuses. AJR 1999; 172: 1535–1540

Definition

▶ **Epidemiology**
More common in women ● Onset is usually at age 25–30 years ● Rare in children and adolescents ● About 20% of patients with stones develop symptoms within 20 years.

▶ **Etiology, pathophysiology, pathogenesis**
Over 90% of cases are due to gallstones ● Secondary bacterial colonization can be found in 70% of cases ● Stoneless forms due to ischemia and secondary infection can occur, especially in intensive care patients ● Opportunistic gallbladder infections occur in immunocompromised patients.

Imaging Signs

▶ **Modality of choice**
Ultrasound ● CT when complications are present.

▶ **Pathognomonic findings**
Thickening of the gallbladder wall in cholelithiasis ● Impacted concretion in the infundibulum of the gallbladder ● Gallbladder is enlarged and more rounded in shape ● Wall is intact in uncomplicated cases ● Gangrenous inflammation produces irregular thickening of the wall ● Wall is often thin in acalculous cases. ● Perforation leads to abscesses in the immediate vicinity ● Gas is present in the wall in emphysematous cholecystitis (infection by gas-forming pathogens).

▶ **Ultrasound findings**
Generalized thickening of the wall (> 4 mm) ● Often several layers of the wall are detectable ● Gallbladder is very tender on palpation (Murphy sign) ● Membranes and echogenic material are present in the lumen ● Fluid is present around the gallbladder.

▶ **CT findings**
Circumscribed or generalized thickening of the wall ● Edema or fluid around the gallbladder, which is usually enlarged ● Wall shows increased enhancement with contrast ● Abscesses in the wall ● Inflammation may spread to the liver ● Where the process has eroded into the duodenum or colon, findings include gas in the collapsed gallbladder and in the bile ducts ● Where large gallstones have eroded into the bowel, findings may include obstructing concretion in the terminal ileum (gallstone ileus).

▶ **MRI findings**
Edema is seen on T2-weighted images as a hyperintensity around the gallbladder ● The gallbladder wall enhances after contrast administration.

▶ **Nuclear medicine studies**
No longer used.

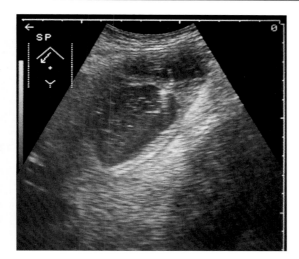

Fig. 2.10 Acute cholecystitis. Ultrasound. Thickened, multilayered gallbladder wall with gallbladder empyema.

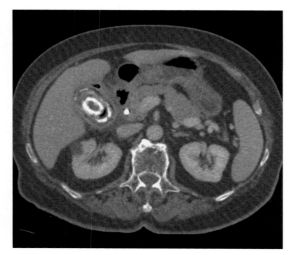

Fig. 2.11 Acute cholecystitis. CT. Perforation into the duodenum (air in the gallbladder lumen).

Clinical Aspects

▸ **Typical presentation**
  Acute persistent or colicky pain in the right upper abdomen ● Nausea, vomiting, and slight fever ● Gallbladder region is very tender to palpation ● Laboratory parameters of inflammation are increased.
▸ **Therapeutic options**
  Antibiotics ● Early elective cholecystectomy.
▸ **Course and prognosis**
  Clinical course is usually uncomplicated ● Acute inflammation lasts about a week ● About one-third of untreated patients have complications; mortality is less than 1%.
▸ **What does the clinician want to know?**
  Cause of the upper abdominal pain and severity of the acute inflammation.

Differential Diagnosis

Kidney stones	– Concretions in the renal calices, renal pelvis, or urinary tract, possibly with obstruction to urine flow
Acute pancreatitis	– Peripancreatic fluid collections
Diverticulitis on the right side	– Circumscribed thickening of the colon wall and pericolic inflammation and/or abscess

Tips and Pitfalls

Can be mistaken for a gallbladder tumor.

Selected Literature

Bennett GL et al. Ultrasound and CT evaluation of emergent gallbladder pathology. Radiol Clin North Am 2003; 41: 1203–1216

Gore RM et al. Imaging benign and malignant disease of the gallbladder. Radiol Clin North Am 2002; 40: 1307–1323

Yusoff IF et al. Diagnosis and management of cholecystitis and cholangitis. Gastroenterol Clin North Am 2003; 32: 1145–1168

Definition

▶ **Epidemiology**
Fifth most common tumor of the gastrointestinal tract • Rare in younger people • Patients are usually over 50 years • Occurs three to five times more often in women • Incidental finding in 1–3 % of all cholecystectomies.

▶ **Etiology, pathophysiology, pathogenesis**
Risk is increased in "porcelain" gallbladder and chronic inflammation with gallstones • Spreads early to the liver, bile duct, and regional lymph nodes.

Imaging Signs

▶ **Modality of choice**
CT, ultrasound.

▶ **Pathognomonic findings**
The gallbladder wall is irregularly and eccentrically thickened • Intraluminal mass • Infiltrative growth in the liver • Enlarged lymph nodes • Cholestasis in the intrahepatic bile ducts.

▶ **Ultrasound findings**
Gallstones are usually present • Irregularly thickened wall • Generally hyperechoic intraluminal mass without an acoustic shadow or a hypoechoic tumor spreading into the liver • The gallbladder wall can be difficult to evaluate when the gallbladder is full of stones.

▶ **CT findings**
Irregular intraluminal polypoid mass that enhances with contrast or a hypodense mass in the bed of the gallbladder that spreads by extension into the hepatic parenchyma • Shows only slight enhancement after contrast administration.

▶ **MRI findings**
Hypointense on T1-weighted images or nearly isointense to the hepatic parenchyma • Hyperintense on T2-weighted images with an ill-defined border along the liver • Heterogeneous enhancement after contrast administration • Infiltration of adjacent organs and lymph node metastases are often easier to evaluate with fat suppression.

▶ **ERCP and PTC**
Now only used for bile duct stenting.

Clinical Aspects

▶ **Typical presentation**
The growing carcinoma remains asymptomatic for a long time • Advanced tumors cause jaundice with or without abdominal pain, loss of appetite, and weight loss • Palpable resistance in the right upper abdomen.

▶ **Therapeutic options**
Resection • Total resection is possible in less than 10% of cases • Extensive tumors require a stent via a transpapillary or percutaneous transhepatic approach.

Fig. 2.12 a, b Gallbladder carcinoma. MR image. Even on the unenhanced scan (**a**), nodular infiltration into the hepatic parenchyma is visible anterior to the gallbladder (arrows). After contrast administration (**b**), the lesion is better differentiated from surrounding liver tissue.

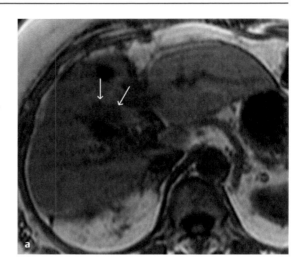

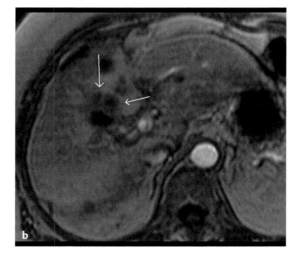

▶ **Course and prognosis**
Five-year survival rate is 5–13 % ● Mean survival time is about 6 months from the diagnosis.

▶ **What does the clinician want to know?**
Infiltration of the liver and lymph node involvement.

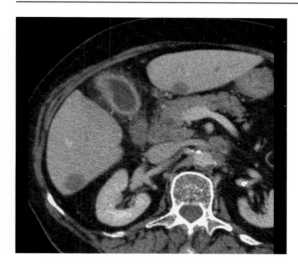

Fig. 2.13 Gallbladder carcinoma. CT. Grossly irregular thickening of the gallbladder wall with patchy infiltration into the surrounding tissue. Other findings include liver metastases and lymph node metastases anterior to the left renal vein.

Differential Diagnosis

Chronic cholecystitis	– Generally uniform thickening of the wall with stones – Homogeneous enhancement
Adenomyomatosis	– Circumscribed or diffuse thickening of the wall with smooth outer contours – Intramural diverticula (Rokitansky–Aschoff sinuses)
Gallbladder polyps	– Cholesterol polyps are usually smaller than 10 mm – Adenomas are usually smaller than 2 cm

Tips and Pitfalls

Can be misdiagnosed as chronic cholecystitis.

Selected Literature

Kalra N, et al. MDCT in the staging of gallbladder carcinoma. AJR 2006; 186: 758–762

Levy AD et al. Gallbladder carcinoma: radiologic-pathologic correlation. RadioGraphics 2001; 21: 295–314

Yun EJ. Gallbladder carcinoma and chronic cholecystitis: differentiation with two-phase spiral CT. Abdom Imaging 2003; 29: 102–108

Definition

Congenital aneurysmal dilatation of any portion of the bile ducts.

▶ **Epidemiology**
Rare developmental anomaly ● Three to four times more common in females ● Higher incidence in Asia ● 80% of cases are diagnosed in children.

▶ **Etiology, pathophysiology, pathogenesis**
Occasionally associated with anomalous pancreaticoduodenal fusion (long common channel over 1.5 cm in length) ● Reflux of bile into the bile duct.
The Todani classification identifies 5 types:

– *Type I:* Fusiform dilation of the extrahepatic bile duct (80–90% of all cases).
– *Type II:* Supraduodenal diverticulum on the extrahepatic bile duct.
– *Type III:* Diverticulum at the level of the duodenal wall (choledochocele).
– *Type IV:* Fusiform dilation of the extrahepatic bile duct with dilation of intrahepatic bile duct segments.
– *Type V:* Cystic dilation of intrahepatic bile ducts (Caroli syndrome).

Imaging Signs

▶ **Modality of choice**
Ultrasound, MRI (including MRCP).

▶ **Pathognomonic findings**
Saccular dilation of the extrahepatic and intrahepatic bile ducts without distal obstruction ● Caroli syndrome involves exclusively the intrahepatic bile ducts ● Intraductal stones with signs of cholangitis ● Bile duct carcinoma is associated with irregular thickening of the bile duct wall and biliary obstruction.

▶ **Ultrasound findings**
Cystic dilation of the bile duct (earliest diagnosis at 25 weeks of pregnancy).

▶ **MRI with MRCP**
Cystic bile duct dilation ● Gallbladder is well demarcated ● Exact extent of the cyst can be determined ● Anomalous pancreaticoduodenal fusion is well visualized.

▶ **Thin-slice CT (with reconstructions) findings**
Cystic bile duct dilation as on MRI.

▶ **ERCP or PTC findings**
Clearly demonstrates the anomaly. Rarely indicated due to the invasive nature of the procedure.

Clinical Aspects

▶ **Typical presentation**
Pain in the right upper abdomen ● Cholangitis ● Jaundice ● Palpable mass.

▶ **Therapeutic options**
Resection and biliodigestive anastomosis.

▶ **Course and prognosis**
Increased risk of infection, stone formation, and bile duct carcinoma.

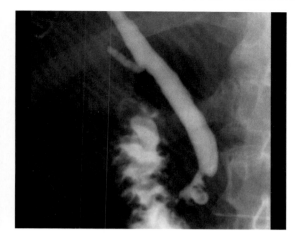

Fig. 2.14 Choledochal cyst. ERCP. Outpouching of the distal bile duct resembling a diverticulum (choledochocele).

► **What does the clinician want to know?**
Exclude an obstructive disorder such as tumor or stones as the cause of the bile duct dilation • Complications develop in cases diagnosed later.

Differential Diagnosis
. . . .

Bile duct tumor	– Dilation of extrahepatic and intrahepatic bile ducts
	– Visible mass
Cholangitis	– Usually associated with gallstones
	– Usually associated with stricture and proximal dilatation
Hepatic and pancreatic cysts	– Round shape
	– Do not communicate with the biliary system
Double gallbladder	– Cystic duct detected
	– Type II is indistinguishable

Tips and Pitfalls
. . . .

Can be confused with biliary obstruction or cysts.

Selected Literature

Irie H et al. Value of MR cholangiopancreatography in evaluating choledochal cysts. AJR 1998; 71: 1381–1385

Matos C et al. Choledochal cyst: comparison of findings at MR cholangiopancreatography and ERCP in eight patients. Radiology 1998; 209: 443–448

Sugiyama M et al. Anomalous pancreatobiliary junction shown on multidetector CT. AJR 2003; 180: 173–175

Todani T et al. Congenital bile duct cysts. Am J Surg 1977; 134: 263–269

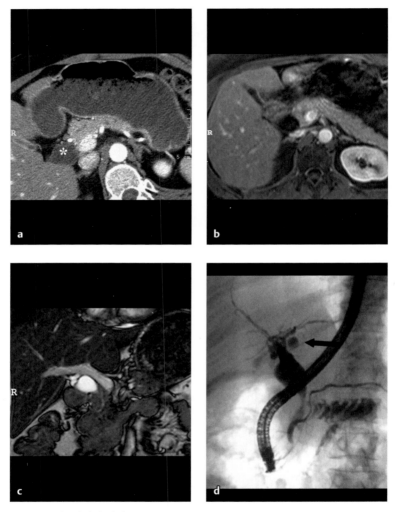

Fig. 2.15 a–d Choledochal cyst.
a CT. Dilated common bile duct.
b T1-weighted MR image. Cystic, dilated hypointense common bile duct.
c T2-weighted MR image. Dilated hyperintense common bile duct.
d ERCP. Saccular outpouching of the proximal common bile duct with a long common channel. Other findings include a second gallbladder arising from the left hepatic duct (arrow).

Definition

Chronic cholestatic liver disorder leading to progressive fibrotic obliteration of the bile ducts.

▶ **Epidemiology**
Fifty to 70 percent of patients are men ● Average age is 40 years.

▶ **Etiology, pathophysiology, pathogenesis**
The etiology is unknown. Immunologic mechanisms play a decisive role, leading to an inflammatory fibrosing process affecting the intrahepatic and extrahepatic ducts ● Often associated with chronic inflammatory bowel disease (70–80% of cases). 2–4% of patients with ulcerative colitis and 1–3% of patients with Crohn disease develop primary sclerosing cholangitis.

Imaging Signs

▶ **Modality of choice**
MRCP, ERCP.

▶ **Pathognomonic findings**
Irregular short and long biliary strictures interspersed with normal or slightly dilated ducts produce a picture resembling a string of pearls ● Outpouchings resembling diverticula and measuring 1–2 mm in diameter occur in 25% of cases ● Obliteration of intrahepatic bile ducts leads to a rarefied biliary system resembling a pruned tree ● Nodular mural irregularities ● Cholelithiasis is present in up to 20–30% of cases ● *Complications:* Biliary cirrhosis (50%) ● Bile duct carcinoma (10–15%) ● Carcinoma of the colon.

▶ **ERCP findings**
Still the gold standard ● Demonstrates early contour irregularities with beginning strictures.

▶ **MRCP findings**
Its limited resolution makes this modality less sensitive than ERCP in diagnosing early stages of the disorder ● In advanced cases, it better visualizes severe intrahepatic pathology, especially proximal to high-grade strictures ● Well suited for follow-up examinations.

▶ **MRI and CT findings**
Concentric or eccentric thickening of the extrahepatic bile duct walls ● Increased contrast enhancement ● Irregularly dilated intrahepatic bile duct segments, some lacking communication with the biliary system ● Fibrosis and cirrhosis.

▶ **Ultrasound findings**
Thickened and hyperechoic bile duct wall.

▶ **Intraductal ultrasound findings**
Irregular thickening of the bile duct wall, occasionally with multiple layers.

Fig. 2.16 a, b Irregular contour and dilation of the intrahepatic bile ducts on ERCP (**a**) and on MRCP (**b**).

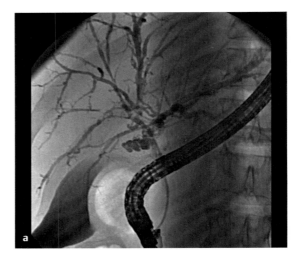

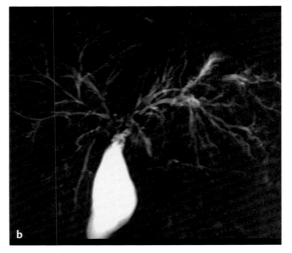

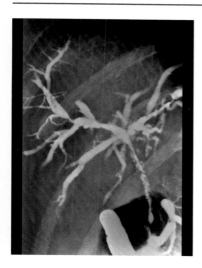

Fig. 2.17 Advanced primary sclerosing cholangitis. ERCP. Intramural diverticulum in the common bile duct and alternating strictures and dilations in the intrahepatic bile ducts.

Clinical Aspects

▶ **Typical presentation**

Onset is insidious with itching, fatigue, jaundice, and fever • Hepatosplenomegaly • Hyperpigmentation • Alkaline phosphatase is 3–10 times normal in 95% of patients • Serum immunoglobulins are raised in up to 80% of patients.

▶ **Therapeutic options**

Ursodeoxycholic acid treatment slows progression of the disorder, reduces the frequency of complications, and also appears to prevent development of carcinomas • Transpapillary balloon dilation and stent implantation are indicated when biliary strictures predominate • Liver transplantation is the only curative treatment for late-stage disease.

▶ **Course and prognosis**

Chronic progressive course culminating in biliary cirrhosis • Development of bile duct carcinoma (annual risk 0.5–1.5%) • Good prognostic models do not yet exist • Mean survival time from diagnosis to death or liver transplantation is 18 years.

▶ **What does the clinician want to know?**

Detection of early-stage primary sclerosing cholangitis • Development of cirrhosis with portal hypertension • Development of bile duct carcinoma.

Differential Diagnosis

Secondary cholangitis	– Medical history (iatrogenic trauma in cholecystectomy, gallstones)
Primary biliary cirrhosis	– Bile ducts are of normal caliber – Impression of the bile ducts by cirrhotic nodules
Bile duct carcinoma	– Circumscribed bile duct wall thickening with dilation – In primary sclerosing cholangitis a developing tumor is difficult to detect on CT and MR images
AIDS cholangiography	– Medical history of HIV infection – Stricture of the distal bile duct often present – Thickening of the gallbladder wall without stones

Tips and Pitfalls

MRCP findings may be equivocal in early-stage disease.

Selected Literature

Fulcher AS et al. Primary sclerosing cholangitis: evaluation with MR cholangiography—a case control study. Radiology 2000; 215: 71–80

Talwalkar J et al. Primary sclerosing cholangitis. Inflamm Bowel Dis 2005; 11: 62–72

Vitellas KM et al. Radiologic manifestations of sclerosing cholangitis with emphasis on MR cholangiopancreatography. RadioGraphics 2000; 20: 959–975

Definition

Malignant tumor of the extrahepatic biliary system with jaundice.

► **Epidemiology**

Seventy to 80 percent of bile duct carcinomas arise in the extrahepatic system •
Rare in younger people • Usually occur at age 50–60 years • Slightly more common in men.

► **Etiology, pathophysiology, pathogenesis**

Incidence is higher in primary sclerosing cholangitis, in congenital biliary
anomalies, and in Asia after infection with *Clonorchis* • Almost exclusively adenocarcinomas • Three forms of growth—nodular exophytic, periductal infiltrative, and intraductal polypoid (rare) • Metastasizes to the lymph nodes • Often
occurs at the bifurcation of the hepatic duct (Klatskin tumor):

– *Type I:* Between the bifurcation of the hepatic duct and the cystic duct.
– *Type II:* At the bifurcation of the hepatic duct without involvement of the right
  or left hepatic duct.
– *Type III:* With involvement of the right or left hepatic duct.
– *Type IV:* Spread to further peripheral bile duct segments.

Imaging Signs

► **Modality of choice**

MRI with MRCP, CT.

► **Pathognomonic findings**

Cholestasis • A small tumor is often present with eccentric or concentric thickening of the wall • Lymph nodes are enlarged in 75% of all cases • Lobar or segmental atrophy that extends into the segment of an intrahepatic bile duct • Infiltration of the liver and vascular structures (sign of irresectability).

► **MRI findings**

On T1-weighted images, the thickened tumorous wall shows slightly decreased
signal intensity or a signal nearly isointense to the hepatic parenchyma • T2-weighted images and MRCP demonstrate narrowing of the bile duct lumen with
peripheral dilation • Usually enhances late after contrast administration • Often
more clearly demarcated with fat suppression • Usually clearly demarcated
against hepatic parenchyma on T2-weighted sequences after SPIO administration.

► **CT findings**

The exact level of the occlusion and the obstructive tumor can usually be well
visualized using thin slices and multiplanar reconstructions • After contrast administration there is usually slight enhancement; occasionally in late phases (5–
10 minutes) there is marked enhancement • Usually the tumor is poorly differentiated from hepatic parenchyma making it difficult to determine the extent of
infiltration in the liver.

Gallbladder and Biliary Tract

Fig. 2.18 Bile duct carcinoma. Ultrasound. A mass is detected in the hilum of the liver with an ill-defined border to the adjacent normal hepatic parenchyma. The bile ducts converge toward the lesion in a stellate pattern and end abruptly.

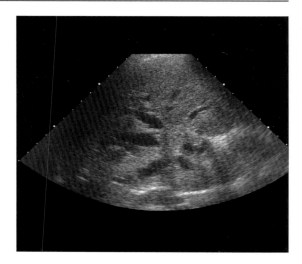

▶ **Ultrasound findings**
Demonstrates the level of the obstruction ● The tumor itself can be visualized in 30–80% of cases as a hypoechoic mass ● In the bifurcation of the hepatic duct, it is difficult to distinguish the lesion from liver tissue.

▶ **Endosonographic findings**
In distal bile duct carcinoma, this modality visualizes the tumor and adjacent lymph nodes and vascular structures at very high resolution.

▶ **ERCP and PTC**
Only indicated for interventional bile duct drainage.

Clinical Aspects

▶ **Typical presentation**
Painless jaundice ● Loss of appetite ● Weight loss.

▶ **Therapeutic options**
Resection ● Extensive tumors are treated with a stent via a transpapillary or percutaneous transhepatic approach ● Photodynamic therapy.

▶ **Course and prognosis**
Five-year survival rate is 0–30% ● Mean survival time is 1 year ● 25% of tumors are resectable ● Mean survival time after resection is 20 months.

▶ **What does the clinician want to know?**
Exclude other benign causes of biliary obstruction (strictures, stones) ● Resectability.

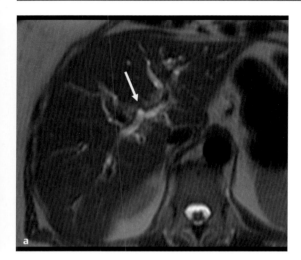

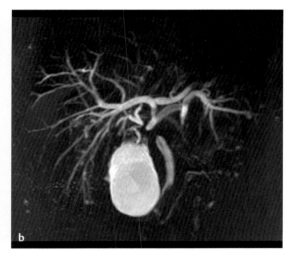

Fig. 2.19 a, b Bile duct carcinoma.
a T2-weighted MR image. Right hepatic duct ends abruptly in the center (arrow).
b MRCP. The tumor obstructs the common hepatic duct and extends on the right to the secondary bifurcation of the bile ducts (type III), whereas the left bile duct is not yet involved.

Differential Diagnosis

Benign stricture	– Obstruction covers a shorter segment – Less severe cholestasis – Less severe wall thickening – Lesser contrast enhancement in the stenoses
Pancreatic carcinoma	– with obstruction of the pancreatic duct – Hypovascular lesion in the head of the pancreas
Bile duct stone	– Intraductal filling defect
Primary sclerosing cholangitis	– Bile ducts resemble a string of pearls

Tips and Pitfalls

After stent placement or drainage, bile duct walls show increased enhancement from inflammation that is practically indistinguishable from tumor proliferation (wherever possible, CT or MR images should be obtained prior to drainage procedures).

Selected Literature

Choi SH et al. Differentiating malignant from benign common bile duct stricture with multiphasic helical CT. Radiology 2005; 236: 178–183

Soto JA et al. Biliary obstruction: findings at MR cholangiography and cross sectional MR imaging. RadioGraphics 2000; 20: 353–366

Soyer P. Imaging of intrahepatic cholangiocarcinoma: hilar cholangiocarcinoma. AJR 1995; 165: 1433–1436

Definition

Congenital anomaly resulting from failure of fusion of the pancreatic ducts.
► **Epidemiology**
  Most common developmental anomaly of the pancreas (3–7% of the population) • No sex predilection.
► **Etiology, pathophysiology, pathogenesis**
  Failure of fusion of the dorsal and ventral buds of the pancreas • The small ventral duct enters the major papilla and the large dorsal duct drains through the
  minor papilla • This results in relative obstruction and increased susceptibility
  to recurrent pancreatitis • *Two forms:* Complete separation and incomplete separation in which the two duct systems communicate via a collateral branch
  (overflow valve).

Imaging Signs

► **Modality of choice**
  MRCP.
► **Pathognomonic findings**
  The main pancreatic duct opens into the minor papilla • The short pancreatic
  duct (which resembles a Bonsai version of a normal pancreatic duct) enters the
  major papilla together with the bile duct • Occasionally the head of the pancreas
  is enlarged and bulky.
► **MRCP findings**
  The main pancreatic duct crosses the distal part of the bile duct • Intravenous
  secretin is recommended to achieve adequate filling of the pancreatic duct.
► **CT findings**
  Where thin slices are used, the course of the main pancreatic duct to the minor
  papilla can usually be delineated on perpendicular reconstructions.
► **ERCP findings**
  Indicated as a purely diagnostic procedure only in exceptional cases • Misinter-
  pretation as abruptly ending duct can result in over-injection of contrast material (with parenchymography).

Clinical Aspects

► **Typical presentation**
  Recurrent abdominal pain (due to the obstruction when the pancreas is stimu-
  lated following consumption of fatty meals or alcohol) • Recurrent pancreatitis • Also occurs as a normal anatomic variant without clinical symptoms (probably the largest group).
► **Therapeutic options**
  Symptomatic cases are treated by sphincterotomy of the minor papilla.

Pancreas

Fig. 3.1 Pancreas divisum. ERCP. The dorsal duct of the pancreas enters the minor papilla. The short ventral pancreatic duct enters the major papilla.

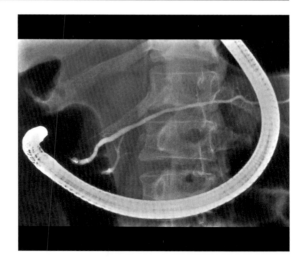

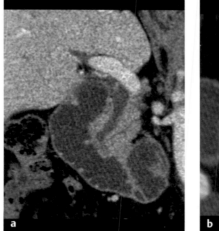

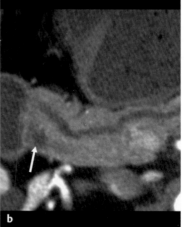

Fig. 3.2 a, b Pancreas divisum. CT.
a The bile duct and the narrow pancreatic duct share a common orifice.
b Perpendicular reconstruction. The pancreatic duct has its own orifice in the minor papilla above the bile duct (arrow).

▶ **Course and prognosis**
Benign disorder with increased risk of pancreatitis.
▶ **What does the clinician want to know?**
Presence of a separate drainage of the pancreatic ducts • Signs of chronic obstructive pancreatitis.

Differential Diagnosis

Pancreatic carcinoma	– Width of the pancreatic duct is normal until interruption by tumor
	– Parenchymal lesion with diminished contrast enhancement

Tips and Pitfalls

Using ERCP as the primary diagnostic modality.

Selected Literature

Matos et al. Pancreas divisum: evaluation with secretin-enhanced magnetic resonance cholangiopancreatography. Gastrointest Endosc 2001; 53: 728–733

Morgan DE et al. Pancreas divisum: implications for diagnostic and therapeutic pancreatography. AJR 1999; 173: 193–198

Soto JA et al. Pancreas divisum: depiction with multi-detector row CT. Radiology 2005; 235: 503–508

Definition

Developmental anomaly leading to duodenal stenosis.

▶ **Epidemiology**
Very rare • No sex predilection.

▶ **Etiology, pathophysiology, pathogenesis**
Defective rotation of the pancreas primordium during embryogenesis • This causes pancreatic tissue to completely or partially encircle the duodenum.
- *Infantile form:* Signs of duodenal stenosis within the first 7 days of life (accounts for 10% of duodenal obstructions).
- *Adult form:* Duodenal stenosis usually develops between the ages of 20 and 30 years as a result of chronic pancreatitis in the glandular ring or due to duodenal ulcerations.

Imaging Signs

▶ **Modality of choice**
MRCP.

▶ **Pathognomonic findings**
Stenosis of the duodenal lumen with normal mucosal surface • Pancreatic tissue or pancreatic duct encircles the duodenum • Occasionally chronic pancreatitis (pseudocysts).

▶ **MRCP findings**
Circular course of the pancreatic duct in the duodenal wall • Secretin should be administered intravenously to ensure sufficient filling of the pancreatic duct.

▶ **CT findings**
Thin CT sections show a uniformly thickened duodenal wall surrounded by a ring of pancreatic parenchyma.

▶ **ERCP findings**
No longer indicated for purely diagnostic purposes • The annular duct segment is only successfully visualized in 50% of cases.

▶ **Findings on upper gastrointestinal series**
Smooth mucosal surface in the region of the obstruction.

▶ **Findings on plain abdominal radiography**
"Double bubble" sign in newborns.

▶ **Ultrasound findings**
When the duodenum is filled with water a ring of pancreatic parenchyma in the duodenal wall will occasionally be detected.

Clinical Aspects

▶ **Typical presentation**
Postprandial vomiting in newborns • Adults have symptoms of chronic pancreatitis or duodenal obstruction.

▶ **Therapeutic options**
High-grade obstruction is treated by duodenojejunal anastomosis.

Pancreas

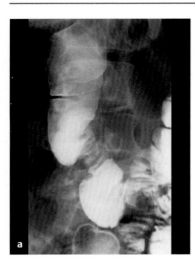

Fig. 3.3 a, b   Annular pancreas.
a Upper gastrointestinal series. Eccentric constriction of the duodenum with intact mucosal contours.
b ERCP. This constriction is due to the annular duct.

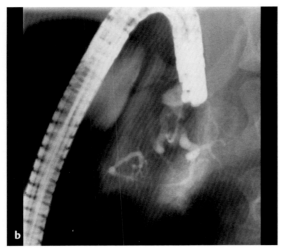

Fig. 3.4 a, b Annu-
lar pancreas. CT.
a A relatively wide
cuff of pancreatic
parenchyma sur-
rounds the duode-
num (star). The an-
nular portion of the
duct is barely visible
(arrow).
b Adjacent imaging
plane. Opening of
the main pancreatic
duct (arrow).

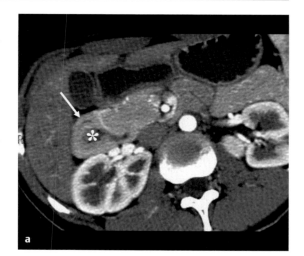

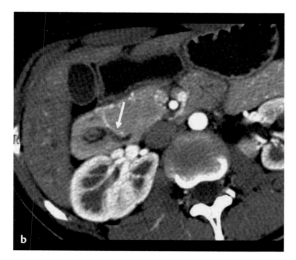

▶ **Course and prognosis**
Benign disorder • Increased risk of chronic pancreatitis.
▶ **What does the clinician want to know?**
Exclude an obstructive tumor of the duodenum.

Differential Diagnosis
....

Duodenal carcinoma	– Irregular thickening of the wall
	– Macroscopic evidence of tumor with endoscopy
Duodenal web	– Thin fold constricting the duodenum

Tips and Pitfalls
....

Can be confused with an obstructive tumor of the duodenum.

Selected Literature

Brambs HJ et al. Diagnostic value of ultrasound in duodenal stenosis. Gastrointest Radiol 1986; 11: 135–139

Jadvar H et al. Annular pancreas in adults: imaging features in seven patients. Abdom Imaging 1999; 24: 174–177

Lecesne R et al. MR cholangiopancreatography of annular pancreas. J Comput Assist Tomogr 1998; 22: 85–86

Definition

Fibrosis and fatty replacement of the normal pancreatic parenchyma due to a hereditary defect of mucus secretion that leads to ductal obstruction.

▶ **Epidemiology**
Most common fatal autosomal recessive disorder in Caucasians • Prevalence is 1:2000–2500 • Most common cause of pancreatic insufficiency before the age of 30 years • Microscopic changes are detectable at birth, macroscopic changes only after 2–3 years.

▶ **Etiology, pathophysiology, pathogenesis**
Defective secretion with increased viscosity of mucus in the bronchi, pancreatic duct and other mucus-producing tissues • The hyperviscosity of the mucus leads to morphologic changes in the lungs and pancreas (obstruction of the pancreatic duct) • Fatty replacement of glandular tissue occurs during the late stages of the disorder.

Imaging Signs

▶ **Modality of choice**
Ultrasound, MRI with MRCP.

▶ **Pathognomonic findings**
Usually fatty replacement of glandular tissue (occasionally with pseudohypertrophy) • Less often fibrosis of the parenchyma (atrophy) • Occasionally small pseudocysts are present • Calcifications are rare (< 10% of cases) • *Extrapancreatic findings:* Periportal fat accumulation, splenomegaly, irregular shape and structure of the liver, small gallbladder with thickened wall and gallstones.

▶ **Ultrasound findings**
Increased echogenicity of the parenchyma • Cysts of varying size are present but large cysts are rare • Often the duct cannot be visualized • Poor correlation between ultrasound findings and gland function.

▶ **MRI with MRCP**
Fatty replacement appears homogeneously hyperintense on T1-weighted images, occasionally showing remnants of lobular architecture • Fibrosis is hypointense on T1-weighted and T2-weighted images • Usually the pancreatic duct cannot be visualized • MRI findings correlate relatively well with function.

▶ **CT findings**
Fatty replacement of pancreatic parenchyma with remnants of lobular architecture.

Clinical Aspects

▶ **Typical presentation**
Clinical manifestation is variable depending on the severity of the disorder and the age of the patient • Meconium ileus occurs in children • Symptoms of chronic bronchitis predominate in older patients • The severity of pancreatic in-

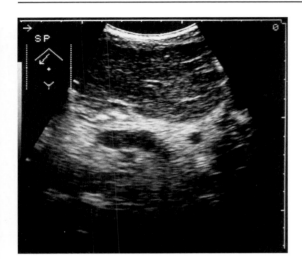

Fig. 3.5 Adolescent patient with cystic fibrosis. Ultrasound. Markedly hyperechoic pancreatic parenchyma.

volvement is variable • Variable pancreatic insufficiency with failure to thrive, steatorrhea, abdominal pain, flatulence.

► **Therapeutic options**
Symptomatic treatment of pancreatic insufficiency.

► **Course and prognosis**
This depends on lung involvement • Exocrine pancreatic insufficiency is present in 85–90% of cases • Endocrine pancreatic insufficiency is present in 30–50%.

► **What does the clinician want to know?**
Severity of pancreatic involvement.

Differential Diagnosis

Lipomatosis	– Usually in obese patients or diabetics
	– No pulmonary manifestation
	– No retention cysts
Chronic pancreatitis	– Dilated pancreatic duct with calcifications
	– Atrophy, no fatty replacement
	– Large pseudocysts
	– Tendency to develop recurrent pancreatitis
Intraductal papillary mucinous neoplasm	– Dilated pancreatic duct and/or side branches
	– Atrophy, no fatty degeneration

Fig. 3.6 a, b Cystic fibrosis. T2-weighted MR image (**a**). Small pseudocyst in the head of the pancreas. The pancreatic parenchyma is completely replaced by fat. MRCP (**b**). The pancreatic duct is not visualized. Lobulated cyst immediately adjacent to the bile duct.

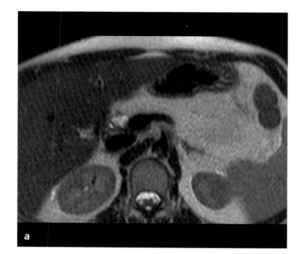

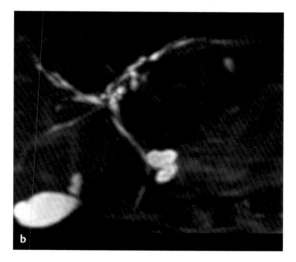

Pancreas

Tips and Pitfalls
. . . .

Can be misinterpreted as lipomatosis when the underlying disorder is not known.

Selected Literature

Ferrozzi F et al. Cystic fibrosis: MR assessment of pancreatic damage. Radiology 1996; 198: 875–879

King LJ et al. Hepatobiliary and pancreatic manifestations of cystic fibrosis: MR imaging appearances. RadioGraphics 2000; 20: 767–777

Soyer P et al. Cystic fibrosis in adolescents and adults: fatty replacement of the pancreas – CT evaluation and functional correlation. Radiology 1999; 210: 611–615

Definition
....

Acute inflammatory process of the pancreas characterized by abdominal pain and raised levels of pancreatic enzymes.

► **Epidemiology**

More common in men ● Usually in young and middle-aged people.

► **Etiology, pathophysiology, pathogenesis**

Most common causes are alcohol misuse and gallstones ● 80–90% of cases have a mild form usually with just exudation and fat necrosis ● A more severe form occurs in 10–20%, with extensive fat necrosis and parenchymal necrosis.

Imaging Signs
....

► **Modality of choice**

In mild cases, ultrasound ● In severe pancreatitis, CT.

► **Pathognomonic findings**

Peripancreatic fluid collections due to exudation, fatty necrosis, and (to a lesser degree) hemorrhage ● Focal or diffuse enlargement of the pancreas ● Parenchymal necrosis showing no perfusion on contrast images ● Pleural effusion is often present (correlating with the severity of the disorder).

Early complications: Infection of the necrotic areas ● Abscesses ● More common in extensive areas of necrosis, where there is a broad area of contact between the necrotic area and the bowel, and in ERCP-induced pancreatitis.

Late complication: Pseudocysts.

► **CT findings**

Peripancreatic fluid collections extending into the retroperitoneum and pararenal space ● Initially there is no border; as time passes a halo of granulation develops ● The extent of parenchymal necrosis can only be estimated after intravenous contrast administration ● Gas is detectable in 20–30% of cases of infected necrosis ● Otherwise CT-guided aspiration is required to demonstrate bacterial contamination.

► **Ultrasound findings**

Gallbladder or bile duct stones can be a sign of biliary pancreatitis ● The extent of peripancreatic fluid collections is more difficult to estimate ● In severe cases, pain and air-filled bowel loops (ileus) interfere with examination.

► **MRI findings**

T2-weighted images provide more information about the composition of peripancreatic fluid collections ● MR cholangiography can demonstrate bile duct stones ● Contrast administration is less of a problem than with CT.

► **ERCP**

Only indicated in severe biliary pancreatitis ● Risk of infection in necrotic areas.

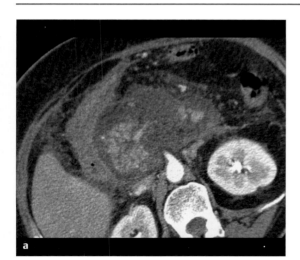

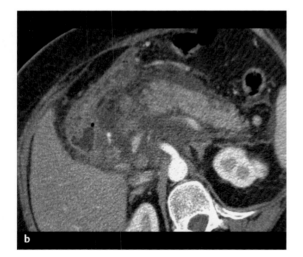

Fig. 3.7 a, b Acute pancreatitis. Extensive peripancreatic exudates. The glandular tissue especially in the head of the pancreas (**a**) is slightly rarefied, probably from fatty tissue necrosis. No major parenchymal defects.

Pancreas

Fig. 3.8 Acute pancreatitis. CT. The air inclusions in the peripancreatic areas of fatty tissue necrosis indicate that they are infected.

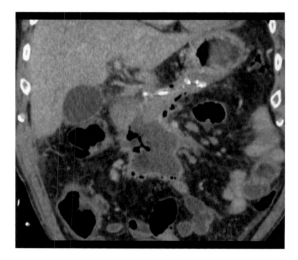

Clinical Aspects

▶ **Typical presentation**
Abdominal pain ● Nausea ● Vomiting ● Fever ● Elevated pancreatic enzymes, leukocytosis, and elevated C-reactive protein (necrosis indicator) ● In the early phases of severe pancreatitis there is an increased risk of multiple organ failure.

▶ **Therapeutic options**
Treatment is primarily conservative ● Antibiotics ● In severe biliary pancreatitis, ERCP with removal of the biliary stones is indicated ● Infected necrotic areas or abscesses often require surgical management or drainage.

▶ **Course and prognosis**
Prognosis is good for mild pancreatitis ● Complications lead to increased morbidity and mortality ● Morbidity and mortality correlate with the extent of extrapancreatic pathology and the extent of parenchymal necrosis (severity index according to Balthazar).

▶ **What does the clinician want to know?**
Extent of necrosis and complications (infection of necrotic areas, abscesses).

Differential Diagnosis

Other causes of acute abdomen	– Pancreas and peripancreatic fatty tissue are normal – CT usually demonstrates another disorder
Chronic pancreatitis	– Atrophic pancreas with dilated duct and calcifications
Lymphoma of the pancreas	– No acute abdomen – Enlarged lymph nodes

Tips and Pitfalls

CT should not be done too early as morphologic changes are fully developed only after 48–72 hours.

Selected Literature

Arvanitakis M et al. Computed tomography and magnetic resonance imaging in the assessment of acute pancreatitis. Gastroenterology 2004; 126: 715

Balthazar EJ. Acute pancreatitis: assessment of severity with clinical and CT evaluation. Radiology 2002; 223: 603–613

Casas JD et al. Prognostic value of CT in the early assessment of patients with acute pancreatitis. AJR 2004; 182: 569–574

Ferrucci JT, Mueller PR. Interventional approach to pancreatic fluid collections. Radiol Clin North Am 2003; 41: 1217–1226

Definition

Persistent inflammation of the pancreas with irreversible morphologic changes usually associated with pain and malabsorption.

▶ **Epidemiology**

Prevalence is 27:100 000 ● Epidemiologic data show considerable geographic variation that is partially attributable to differences in alcohol consumption.

▶ **Etiology, pathophysiology, pathogenesis**

Most common cause is alcohol misuse; it accounts for 70–90% of cases ● However, only 5–15% of heavy drinkers develop chronic pancreatitis ● Smoking appears to promote the development of calcifying pancreatitis ● Other forms are tropical pancreatitis, hereditary forms, metabolic forms, disease from obstructive causes, and idiopathic disease.

Imaging Signs

▶ **Modality of choice**

Ultrasound ● MRCP ● CT where complications are present.

▶ **Pathognomonic findings**

Atrophy of the pancreatic parenchyma ● Irregularly dilated main pancreatic duct and side branches, in advanced disease with intraductal calcifications.
Complications: Pancreas pseudocysts ● Biliary obstruction ● Pseudoaneurysms with hemorrhage ● Splenic vein thrombosis.

▶ **Ultrasound findings**

The parenchyma appears inhomogeneous in early phases and later becomes increasingly atrophic ● Pancreatic duct is dilated; concretions are often present.

▶ **CT findings**

Not suitable for evaluating early forms ● Initially and in acute inflammation, findings include circumscribed or diffuse enlargement of the pancreas ● Later findings include atrophic parenchyma, dilated ducts, and calcifications ● Pseudocysts.

▶ **MRCP findings**

The Cambridge classification (proposed for ERCP) can be applied for moderate and severe forms ● After contrast administration, there is heterogeneous parenchymal enhancement ● Intravenous secretin and oral SPIO allows semiquantitative evaluation of exocrine pancreas function.

▶ **MRI findings**

T1-weighted images show decreasing signal intensity in the parenchyma and decreased contrast enhancement due to fibrosis ● Calcifications are poorly visualized ● On T2-weighted images, acutely inflamed areas, necrotic areas, and pseudocysts appear hyperintense ● Dilated ducts are well visualized on T2-weighted images and MRCP.

▶ **ERCP**

No longer used in primary diagnostics, although it provides the most precise images of ductal changes ● Only important in interventions in the pancreas.

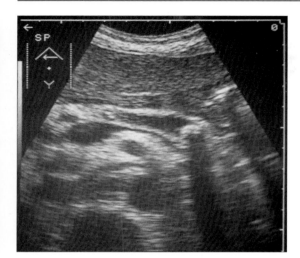

Fig. 3.9 Chronic pancreatitis. Ultrasound. Dilated pancreatic duct with a concretion casting an acoustic shadow. The hyperechoic pancreatic parenchyma is atrophic and narrowed.

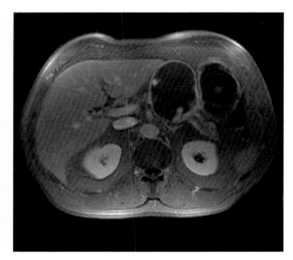

Fig. 3.10 Chronic pancreatitis. T1-weighted MR image after contrast administration. Large pancreatic pseudocyst with an artery projecting into the cystic lumen (risk of hemorrhage from vascular erosion).

▶ **Endosonographic findings**
Most precise visualization of parenchymal and ductal changes in the pancreas ● However, it is easy to overestimate the extent of damage.

▶ **Findings on plain abdominal radiography**
Calcifications projected on the pancreas ● No longer used as a diagnostic modality.

Pancreas

Clinical Aspects

▶ **Typical presentation**
   Pain (most common indication for surgery) ● Weight loss ● Steatorrhea and other signs of malabsorption ● Diabetes mellitus.

▶ **Therapeutic options**
   Surgery is indicated in patients with complications and severe pain ● Endoscopic
   removal of pancreatic duct stones and stenting for stenosis of the distal bile duct
   and of high-grade pancreatic duct strictures.

▶ **Course and prognosis**
   Exocrine and endocrine insufficiency can result in chronic cases ● Mortality is
   primarily influenced by chronic alcohol misuse ● Increased incidence of pancreatic carcinomas.

▶ **What does the clinician want to know?**
   Complications such as pseudocysts, pseudoaneurysm, and ductal obstruction ●
   Exclude pancreatic carcinoma.

Differential Diagnosis

Pancreatic carcinoma	– Parenchymal atrophy and ductal dilation distal to the tumor
	– Signs of infiltration
	– Differential diagnosis can be difficult when areas of acute inflammation are present in chronic pancreatitis
Intraductal papillary mucinous neoplasm	– No history of alcoholism
	– Usually no calcifications
	– Enhancing intraductal polyps
Acute pancreatitis	– Extensive peripancreatic fluid collections
	– No pancreatic atrophy

Tips and Pitfalls

Can be misinterpreted as a pancreatic carcinoma.

Selected Literature

Cappeliez O et al. Chronic pancreatitis: evaluation of pancreatic exocrine function with
   MR pancreatography after secretin stimulation. Radiology 2000; 215: 358–362

Luetmer PH et al. Chronic pancreatitis reassessment with current CT. Radiology 1989;
   171: 353–357

Semelka RC et al. Chronic pancreatitis: MR imaging features before and after administration of gadopentetate dimeglumine. J Magn Reson Imaging 1993; 3: 79–82

Definition

Synonyms: Primary sclerosing pancreatitis, lymphoplasmacytic sclerosing pancreatitis, nonalcoholic chronic pancreatitis with duct destruction. Special form of chronic pancreatitis primarily associated with duct destruction.

▶ **Epidemiology**
Occurs in all age groups ● Slightly more common in men ● According to European and American publications, disease tends to occur in young individuals (35–40 years) ● In Asia, disease often occurs in older patients (60 years).

▶ **Etiology, pathophysiology, pathogenesis**
Pathogenesis is unclear ● Associated with autoimmune disorders in up to 50% of cases ● Presumably a heterogeneous clinical picture ● Distinguished from other forms of chronic pancreatitis by periductal lymphoplasmacytic infiltrates that eventually lead to duct strictures and fibrosis ● Often spreads to the bile duct and can lead to alterations resembling primary sclerosing cholangitis.

Imaging Signs

▶ **Modality of choice**
MRI, CT and ERCP.

▶ **Pathognomonic findings**
Diffuse or circumscribed enlargement of the organ occurs in the active phase ● May develop as a pseudotumor ● Diffuse or segmental stenosis (more than one-third of the length) of the pancreatic duct ● Stenosis of the distal bile duct occurs relatively often, sometimes resembling primary sclerosing cholangitis ● No peripancreatic fluid collections ● Occasionally associated with phlebitis of the splenic vein.

▶ **MRI findings**
Inflamed segment is hyperintense on T2-weighted images ● Relatively uniform but generally reduced contrast enhancement occurs in diffuse involvement ● In circumscribed forms, the affected areas show less enhancement ● Contrast enhancement in the wall of the distal part of the bile duct ● Strictures of the pancreatic duct are not adequately visualized on MRCP ● Intact parenchyma is probably best evaluated after administration of manganese DPDP.

▶ **CT findings**
"Sausage-shaped" pancreas (loss of the usual glandular lobulation) ● Affected areas show less enhancement.

▶ **ERCP findings**
Most detailed visualization of the irregular strictures, which usually occur over a long segment.

▶ **Endosonographic findings**
Focal or diffuse changes in the internal structure of the pancreas ● Probably the best modality for guiding a biopsy.

Pancreas

Fig. 3.11 a–c   Autoimmune pancreatitis.
a   CT, arterial phase.
Slightly swollen pancreas
with narrow rim (arrow).
b   CT. Portal venous
phase. Here, too, there is a
narrow rim around the
slightly swollen pancreas.
Thrombosis of the splenic
vein (arrow).
c   MRI. After administration of manganese DPDP
the areas of intact parenchyma enhance only
slightly and inhomoge-
neously.

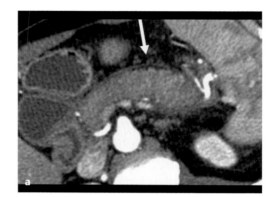

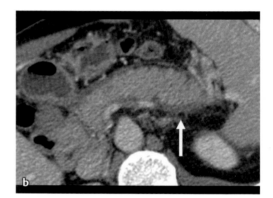

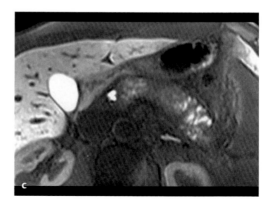

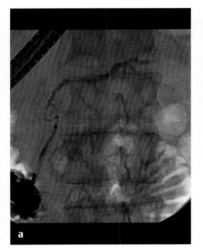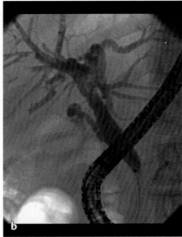

Fig. 3.12 a, b Autoimmune pancreatitis. ERCP.
a Long stenosis of the pancreatic duct in the head and slight dilation in the body.
b Severe stenosis of the distal bile duct.

Clinical Aspects

▶ **Typical presentation**
Slight abdominal symptoms ● European and American publications report mild attacks of acute pancreatitis in 50–75 % of cases, whereas these are rare in Asian studies ● Jaundice occasionally occurs ● Diagnosis is essentially based on radiologic findings and to a lesser extent on laboratory data (raised gammaglobulin and/or immunoglobulin G levels) and histologic findings.

▶ **Therapeutic options**
Steroids.

▶ **Course and prognosis**
The natural course of the disorder is not known ● Symptoms usually improve under steroid therapy.

▶ **What does the clinician want to know?**
Exclude pancreatic carcinoma.

Differential Diagnosis

Pancreatic carcinoma	– Duct is obstructed over a short segment, followed by dilation
	– Tumor usually does not enhance with contrast and infiltrates at an early stage
Chronic pancreatitis	– Duct dilation and calcifications
Acute pancreatitis	– Almost invariably associated with extensive peripancreatic fluid collections

Tips and Pitfalls

Can be misinterpreted as pancreatic carcinoma, leading to unnecessary resection of the pancreas.

Selected Literature

Finkelberg DL et al. Autoimmune pancreatitis. N Engl J Med 2006; 355: 2670–2676

Kawamoto S et al. Lymphoplasmacytic sclerosing pancreatitis with obstructive jaundice: CT and pathology features. AJR 2004; 183: 915–921

Sahani DV et al. Autoimmune pancreatitis: imaging features. Radiology 2004; 233: 345–352

Definition

▶ **Epidemiology**

Most common ductal exocrine tumor of the pancreas • Accounts for 80% of exocrine tumors of the pancreas • Average patient age is 50–70 years • Slightly more common in men.

▶ **Etiology, pathophysiology, pathogenesis**

Extremely aggressive tumor; incidence and mortality are nearly identical • Most often occurs in the head of the pancreas (60% of all lesions).

Imaging Signs

▶ **Modality of choice**

CT (most practical modality for diagnosis, staging, and evaluation of resectability).

▶ **Pathognomonic findings**

Mass with ill-defined margins • Poorly vascularized • Dilation of the pancreatic duct (early sign) and the bile duct (double duct sign) • Chronic ductal obstruction causes parenchymal atrophy • Early infiltration occurs into the retroperitoneal fatty tissue, adjacent vascular structures, and adjacent organs • Liver metastases and lymph node involvement are common.

▶ **CT findings**

The hypovascular tumor is most readily distinguished from the surrounding parenchyma during the parenchymal phase • Obstruction of the pancreatic duct and bile duct is well visualized (rendering ERCP superfluous).

▶ **Ultrasound findings**

Hypoechoic tumor with cholestasis and congestion of the pancreatic duct, usually readily detectable • Liver metastases are usually diagnosed at a very early stage.

▶ **Endosonographic findings**

Good method for local staging • Superior to CT and MRI for small tumors.

▶ **MRI findings**

Hypointense on T1-weighted images with only slight contrast enhancement • Slightly hypointense on T2-weighted images • In combination with MRCP, this modality visualizes the pancreatic duct and bile ducts in sufficient detail • The diagnostic information is about equal to CT, but the technique is more complicated.

▶ **ERCP**

Practically no longer used in diagnosing pancreatic carcinoma; does not provide any useful information on resectability • Indicated for bile duct stenting.

Fig. 3.13 Ductal adenocarcinoma of the pancreas. Hypovascular carcinoma of the tail of the pancreas infiltrating the hilum of the spleen and the stomach.

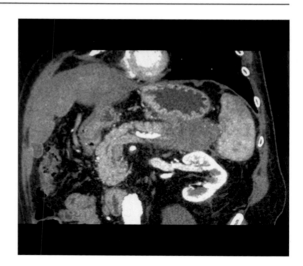

Clinical Aspects

▸ **Typical presentation**
Jaundice • Back pain • Loss of appetite • Weight loss.
▸ **Therapeutic options**
Surgical excision when resectability criteria are fulfilled • Otherwise bile duct stent is indicated.
▸ **Course and prognosis**
Most patients die within 1–2 years of the diagnosis • 5-year survival rate in most studies is no higher than 2–3 %.
▸ **What does the clinician want to know?**
Evaluate resectability • Exclude chronic pancreatitis and other less aggressive tumors.

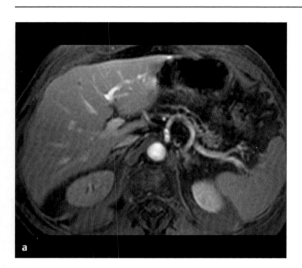

Fig. 3.14 a, b
Ductal adenocarci-
noma of the pan-
creas. MR image.
a Dilation of the
pancreatic duct,
atrophy of the pan-
creatic parenchyma.
b Hypovascular
tumor in the head
of the pancreas.

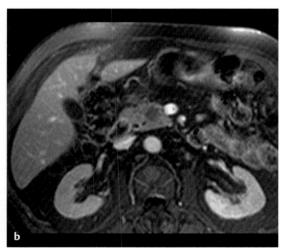

Differential Diagnosis

Chronic pancreatitis	– Chronic alcoholism – Usually generalized enlargement of the pancreas – Parenchymal atrophy – Calcifications
Autoimmune pancreatitis	– Stricture of the pancreatic duct, usually over a long segment – Usually in younger patients – Associated with other autoimmune disorders – Gammaglobulin often elevated
Metastases	– In far advanced stages, usually with a known primary tumor
Endocrine tumors	– Usually hypervascular or with hypervascular components – 30% of nonfunctioning malignant tumors have calcifications
Solid papillary tumor	– Primarily occurs in young women – Usually exhibits cystic components or hemorrhages
Mucinous cystadeno-carcinoma	– Usually more clearly demarcated – Cystic – Calcifications in the cyst wall – Almost exclusively in women

Tips and Pitfalls

Can be misinterpreted as chronic pancreatitis • Lesion should not be assessed as irresectable solely on the basis of vascular infiltration.

Selected Literature

Catalano C et al. Pancreatic carcinoma: the role of high resolution multislice spiral CT in the diagnosis and assessment of resectability. Eur Radiol 2003; 13: 149–156

Fletcher JG et al. Pancreatic malignancy: value of arterial, pancreatic, and hepatic phase imaging with multi-detector row CT. Radiology 2003; 229: 81–90

Nishiharu T et al. Local extension of pancreatic carcinoma: assessment with thin-section helical CT versus breath-hold fast MR imaging—ROC analysis. Radiology 1999; 212: 445–452

Tamm EP et al. Diagnosis, staging, and surveillance of pancreatic cancer. AJR 2003; 180: 1311–1323

Definition

Usually benign primary cystic tumor of the pancreas consisting of multiple small cysts.

▶ **Epidemiology**
Accounts for 1–2% of all exocrine tumors of the pancreas ● Average patient age is 50–70 years ● Considerably more common in women.

▶ **Etiology, pathophysiology, pathogenesis**
Cysts are lined with PAS-positive epithelial cells with high glycogen content that secrete a serous fluid ● Uniformly distributed throughout the pancreas ● Tumor size ranges from 1 cm to 25 cm (average size is 6–11 cm) ● Usually occurs sporadically ● Occurs in 60–80% of patients with von Hippel–Lindau syndrome.

Imaging Signs

▶ **Modality of choice**
CT, MRI.

▶ **Pathognomonic findings**
Well-demarcated tumor comprised of many small cysts (up to 2 cm in size) that resemble a honeycomb or sponge ● Lobulated contour with thin cyst walls that enhance with contrast ● Occasionally there is a stellate scar with central calcifications (20–30% of cases) ● Lesion does not communicate with the pancreatic duct system ● Bile ducts and pancreatic duct are usually not dilated ● A macrocystic (oligocystic) variant occurs in up to 10% of all cases.

▶ **CT findings**
The microcystic structure is usually detectable at high resolution and after intravenous contrast administration.

▶ **MRI findings**
T2-weighted images and MRCP clearly visualize the cystic composition of the tumor. The small cysts are hyperintense and do not communicate with the pancreatic duct system.

▶ **Endosonographic findings**
Allows biopsy and analysis of cyst content—serous fluid, amylase and tumor markers are not elevated.

Clinical Aspects

▶ **Typical presentation**
Usually an incidental finding ● Larger tumors can cause a pressure sensation.

▶ **Therapeutic options**
Surgical removal is indicated when the tumor causes symptoms due to its size.

▶ **Course and prognosis**
Malignant degeneration is very rare ● This justifies follow-up with imaging studies ● Average growth rate is 4 mm per year.

Fig. 3.15a–c   Serous cystadenoma of the pancreas.
a, b CT. Honeycomb pattern of small cysts whose fine walls enhance with contrast.
c Surgical specimen.

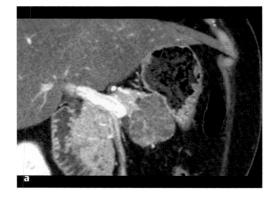

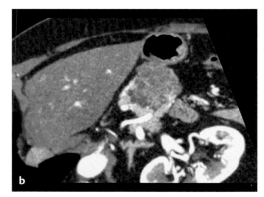

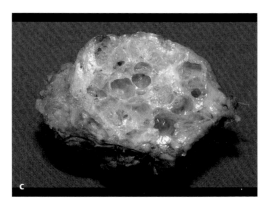

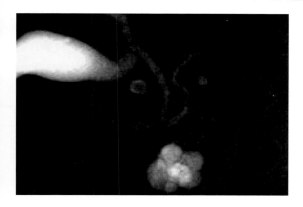

Fig. 3.16 Serous cystadenoma of the pancreas. MRCP. The clustered structure of the cystadenoma resembling a bunch of grapes is clearly seen.

Pancreas

▶ **What does the clinician want to know?**
Distinguish from mucinous cystic tumors (mucinous cystadenoma or cystadeno-carcinoma and intraductal papillary mucinous neoplasm) as these require surgical excision.

Differential Diagnosis

Mucinous cystadenoma	– Large cysts with septa and thickened walls – Cyst walls occasionally contain calcifications – Does not communicate with the duct system – Difficult to distinguish from macrocystic variant
Intraductal papillary mucinous neoplasm	– Side branch lesion can appear similar – Usually does not result in a circumscribed mass – Essentially consists of dilated ducts – No calcifications
Solid papillary tumor	– Primarily occurs in young women – Usually large ill-defined areas of cystic necrosis

Tips and Pitfalls

Can be misinterpreted as mucinous tumor that represents an absolute indication for surgery.

Selected Literature

Cohen-Scali F et al. Discrimination of unilocular macrocystic serous cystadenoma from pancreatic pseudocyst and mucinous cystadenoma with CT: initial observations. Radiology 2003; 228: 727–733

Curry CA et al. CT of primary cystic pancreatic neoplasms. AJR 2000; 175: 99–103

Procacci C et al. Serous cystadenoma of the pancreas: report of 30 cases with emphasis on imaging findings. J Comput Assist Tomogr 1997; 21: 373–382

Definition

Primary cystic tumor of the pancreas with malignant potential consisting of mucus-filled cysts that do not communicate with the pancreatic duct system.

▶ **Epidemiology**

Accounts for 1–2% of all exocrine tumors of the pancreas • Average age is 40–80 years • Occurs almost exclusively in women.

▶ **Etiology, pathophysiology, pathogenesis**

Ovarylike stroma • Lined with mucus-secreting epithelial cells • Classified as adenoma, borderline tumor, or carcinoma depending on the degree of dysplasia • About a third of all lesions are still benign at the time of diagnosis • Usually occur in the body and tail of the pancreas • Size is 2–25 cm (average 6–10 cm).

Imaging Signs

▶ **Modality of choice**

CT, MRI.

▶ **Pathognomonic findings**

Usually comprises several large cysts (> 2 cm) • Well-demarcated tumor with septa • Occasionally there is a thick cyst wall • Does not communicate with the pancreatic duct system • Bile duct and pancreatic duct may be dilated due to compression • Peripheral eggshell calcifications suggest malignancy.

▶ **CT findings**

Tumor made up of large cysts with septa • Cyst wall enhances with contrast.

▶ **MRI findings**

Hyperintense cysts on T2-weighted images and MRCP • Septa are well demarcated • Does not communicate with the pancreatic duct.

▶ **Endosonographic findings**

Allows biopsy and analysis of cyst content—mucinous fluid, with necrosis and hemorrhages. Tumor markers are raised; amylase is not.

Clinical Aspects

▶ **Typical presentation**

Large tumors cause pressure sensation and abdominal pain • Loss of appetite • Weight loss.

▶ **Therapeutic options**

Surgical removal of the benign forms is also indicated as malignant degeneration is common.

▶ **Course and prognosis**

Prognosis is good when complete resection of the tumor is possible (5-year survival rate is > 95%) • In patients younger than 50 years and in those with invasive tumors, prognosis is less favorable.

▶ **What does the clinician want to know?**

Rule out pancreatic pseudocysts • Signs of malignant degeneration.

Pancreas

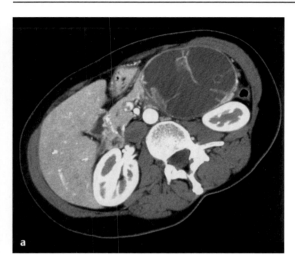

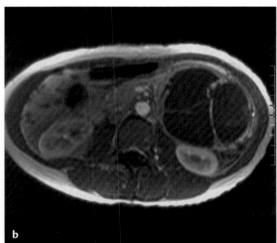

Fig. 3.17 a–d
Mucinous cystade-
noma of the pan-
creas.
a CT, arterial
phase. The fine
septa are well
visualized.
b T1-weighted MR
image after contrast
administration.
Septa are well
visualized.

c   Mucinous cystadenoma. T2-weighted MR image. Cysts contain fluid of varying signal intensity.

d   MRCP. Displacement of the pancreatic duct in the tail, with high signal intensity only in isolated cystic compartments.

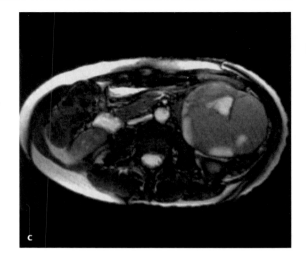

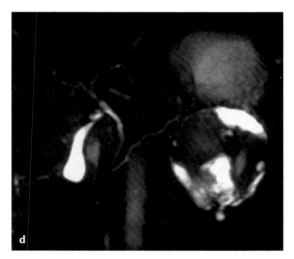

Differential Diagnosis

Pseudocysts	– Sequela of acute or chronic pancreatitis (medical history)
Serous cystadenoma	– Many small cysts in a honeycomb configuration – Central stellate scar and calcifications occasionally present
Intraductal papillary mucinous neoplasm	– Mucus-filled cystic dilated pancreatic ducts – Intraductal polyps
Solid papillary tumor	– Primarily occurs in young women – Solid and cystic components – Hemorrhages
Cystic degenerative tumors	– Infiltrative growth and metastases

Tips and Pitfalls

Can be misinterpreted as a pancreatic pseudocyst, resulting in unnecessary therapeutic cystojejunostomy.

Selected Literature

Brugge WR et al. Cystic neoplasms of the pancreas. N Engl J Med 2004; 16: 1218–1226

Cohen-Scali F et al. Discrimination of unilocular macrocystic serous cystadenoma from pancreatic pseudocyst and mucinous cystadenoma with CT: initial observations. Radiology 2003; 228: 727–733

Sahani V et al. Cystic pancreatic lesions: a simple imaging-based classification system for guiding management. RadioGraphics 2005; 25: 1471–1484

Definition

Primary cystic tumor of the pancreas arising from the ductal epithelium with mucous secretions that lead to dilation of the pancreatic ducts.

▶ **Epidemiology**

Accounts for 1–2% of all exocrine tumors of the pancreas ● Average age is 60–80 years ● Slightly more common in men.

▶ **Etiology, pathophysiology, pathogenesis**

Obstruction by mucus leads to fibrosis and parenchymal atrophy as in chronic pancreatitis.

Three forms: Side branch lesion (predilection for the uncinate process), main duct lesion, and mixed lesion ● Side branch lesions most frequently appear to be benign ● Tumors are classified as benign, borderline, or malignant according to their differentiation ● Carcinoma in situ is present in 7–34% of cases ● Invasive carcinoma is present in 25–44%.

Imaging Signs

▶ **Modality of choice**

CT, MRI.

▶ **Pathognomonic findings**

Cystic dilation of the side branches and/or circumscribed or diffuse dilation of the main duct ● No ductal calcifications ● Small intraductal papillary nodules are present that enhance with contrast ● Mucus plugs are present in the ducts ● Prominent papilla ● A circumscribed tumor mass is usually only detectable in malignant forms ● *Signs of malignancy:* Large nodules on the walls, extremely dilated ducts (> 10 mm), and obstruction of the bile duct ● Vascular infiltration is rare.

▶ **CT findings**

Reconstructions from multidetector CT with thin slices visualizes the communication with the duct ● The intraductal nodules enhance on multiphase CT.

▶ **MRI findings**

T2-weighted images and MRCP show cystic dilatation of the ducts ● Communicates with the duct system ● Unlike ERCP, this modality can distinguish mucus from papillary nodules (intraductal filling voids).

▶ **Endosonographic findings**

Allows biopsy and analysis of cyst content—mucus secretion, raised amylase, raised tumor markers.

▶ **Endoscopy and ERCP findings**

Prominent papilla from which viscous mucus drains ● The mucus can cause filling defects in the pancreatic duct and make it difficult to achieve complete filling of the duct system.

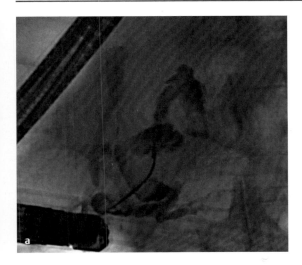

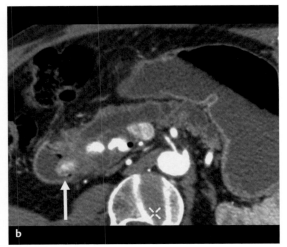

Fig. 3.18 a, b Intraductal papillary mucinous neoplasm of the pancreas.
a ERCP. Incomplete filling of the pancreatic duct, which exhibits a large filling defect in the head caused by mucus.
b CT performed immediately after ERCP. Marked dilation of the main pancreatic duct and atrophy of the pancreatic parenchyma. Residual contrast medium from ERCP is visible in the side branches in the head of the pancreas. Some contrast medium also remains in the prominent papilla (arrow).

Fig. 3.19 a, b Intraductal papillary mucinous neoplasm of the pancreas.
a T2-weighted MR image. The pancreatic duct is greatly dilated in the head and body.
b Marked dilation of the main duct in the head of the pancreas and cystic dilation of the side branches.

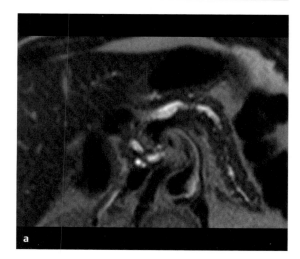

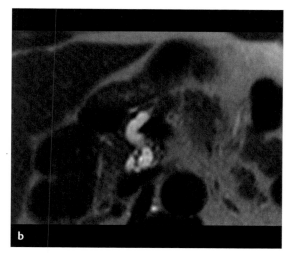

Clinical Aspects

▶ **Typical presentation**
Clinical picture of chronic pancreatitis is often present ● Episodes of mild pancreatitis can occasionally occur.

▶ **Therapeutic options**
Surgical removal.

▶ **Course and prognosis**
Survival is long in the absence of invasive growth ● Prognosis is significantly worse for the malignant variant with lymph node metastases ● The tumor can recur locally as an extrapancreatic lesion (usually solid) or intrapancreatic lesion (usually cystic).

▶ **What does the clinician want to know?**
Extent of ductal involvement as this determines the extent of the resection ● Exclude nonmucinous cystic tumors (serous cystadenoma) as these do not necessarily require resection.

Differential Diagnosis

Chronic pancreatitis	– History of alcoholism
	– Advanced cases can involve calcifications in the parenchyma and ducts
Serous cystadenoma	– Many small cysts in a honeycomb configuration that form a circumscribed tumor
	– Central stellate scar and calcifications often present
	– Does not communicate with the duct system
Mucinous cystadenoma	– Large cysts with septa and thickened walls
	– Cyst walls occasionally contain calcifications
	– Does not communicate with the duct system
	– Almost exclusively in women

Tips and Pitfalls

Can be misinterpreted as chronic pancreatitis.

Selected Literature

Fukukura Y et al. Intraductal papillary mucinous tumors of the pancreas: Comparison of helical CT and MR imaging. Acta Radiol 2003; 44: 464–471

Irie H et al. MR cholangiopancreatographic differentiation of benign and malignant intraductal mucinproducing tumors of the pancreas. AJR 2000; 174: 1403–1408

Kawamoto S et al. Intraductal papillary mucinous neoplasm of the pancreas: Can benign lesions be differentiated from malignant lesions with MDCT? RadioGraphics 2005; 25: 1451–1470

Definition

Moderately malignant tumor of the pancreas with solid and cystic components •
Synonyms: Solid and cystic tumor, papillary cystic tumor.

► **Epidemiology**
Accounts for less than 1% of all exocrine tumors of the pancreas • Occurs almost
exclusively in young women (about age 30 years).

► **Etiology, pathophysiology, pathogenesis**
Consists of solid and cystic components • Necrosis and hemorrhage are typical •
Can arise in every segment of the pancreas, apparently with a slight predilection
for the head • Average size is 9–12 cm.

Imaging Signs

► **Modality of choice**
CT, MRI.

► **Pathognomonic findings**
Large tumor with solid and cystic components • Can also appear completely sol-
id or cystic • Usually with a thick-walled capsule that enhances with contrast •
Calcifications occur in 30% of cases • Signs of hemorrhage are often present •
Does not communicate with the pancreatic duct system • Bile duct and pancre-
atic duct are not dilated because the tumor is soft.

► **CT findings**
Solid components enhance slightly during the arterial phase • Marked enhancement occurs during the portal venous phase.

► **MRI findings**
Hemorrhagic necrotic areas appear hyperintense on T1-weighted images and hypointense on T2-weighted images • Tumor is highly heterogeneous on T2-
weighted images • Layering is occasionally observed • Contrast enhancement
begins early at the periphery and progresses toward the center.

► **Ultrasound findings**
Hemorrhages appear hyperechoic.

► **Endosonographic findings**
Allows biopsy and analysis of cyst content—mucinous fluid, with necrosis and
hemorrhages. Tumor markers are raised; amylase is not.

Clinical Aspects

► **Typical presentation**
Symptoms only occur with large tumors • Pressure sensation • Abdominal
pain • Loss of appetite • Weight loss.

► **Therapeutic options**
Surgical removal.

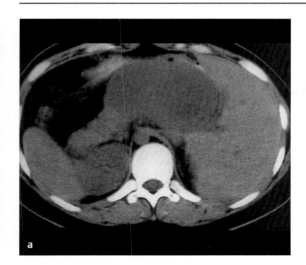

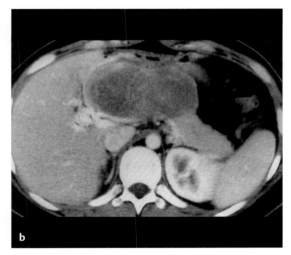

Fig. 3.20 a, b
Solid pseudopapillary tumor. CT.
a Unenhanced scan. Cystic tumor with homogeneous structure in the head of the pancreas.
b After contrast administration. Only slight contrast enhancement, primarily close to the capsule.

Fig. 3.21 a, b Partially cystic, partially solid tumor of the tail of the pancreas that exhibits cystic areas on both CT (**a**) and T2-weighted MR image (**b**) (used with the kind permission of Professor Rieber-Brambs, Munich).

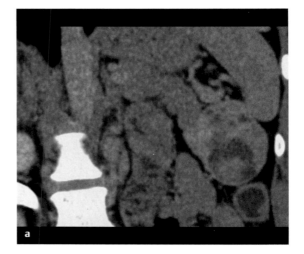

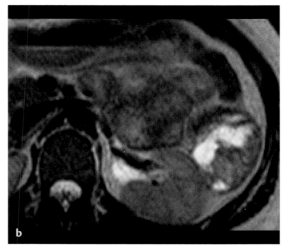

▶ **Course and prognosis**

Prognosis is good where the tumor can be completely resected (> 95% cure rate) ● In a few cases, the course is less favorable due to liver metastases ● Prognosis is less favorable in older patients.

▶ **What does the clinician want to know?**

Exclude pancreatic pseudocysts.

Differential Diagnosis

Pseudocysts	– Sequela of acute or chronic pancreatitis (medical history)
Serous cystadenoma	– Many small cysts in a honeycomb configuration – Central stellate scar and calcifications occasionally present – Does not communicate with the duct system
Mucinous cystadenoma	– Large cysts with septa and thickened walls – Cyst walls occasionally contain calcifications – Does not communicate with the duct system
Cystic degenerative tumors	– Infiltrative growth and metastases
Pancreatoblastoma	– Almost exclusively in children

Tips and Pitfalls

Can be misinterpreted as a traumatic pancreatic pseudocyst.

Selected Literature

Buetow PC et al. Solid and papillary epithelial neoplasm of the pancreas: imaging-pathologic correlation in 56 cases. Radiology 1996; 199: 707–711

Cantisani V et al. MR imaging features of solid pseudopapillary tumor of the pancreas in adult and pediatric patients. AJR 2003; 181: 395–340

Merkle EM et al. Papillary cystic and solid tumor of the pancreas. Z Gastroenterol 1996; 34: 743–746

Definition

Neuroendocrine tumors of the pancreas whose hormone secretions cause specific symptoms.

► **Epidemiology**

Rare tumors ● Most common tumors of this type are insulinoma and gastrinoma with an incidence of 0.3–3/1 000 000 ● Peak age for insulinoma is 30–60 years; women are affected slightly more often ● Peak age for gastrinoma is 30–50 years; men are affected more often.

► **Etiology, pathophysiology, pathogenesis**

Usually occur sporadically ● Can also be associated with genetic syndromes—MEN syndrome, von Hippel—Lindau syndrome, neurofibromatosis, and tuberous sclerosis ● Rate of malignancy varies: Insulinoma 10%, gastrinoma of the pancreas 70%, gastrinoma of the duodenum 40%, VIPoma 50–75%, glucagonoma 65–75% ● Histologic differentiation between benign and malignant tumors is difficult ● *Typical location and size:*

– Insulinoma (1–8 cm) occurs in the pancreas in over 99% of cases.
– Gastrinoma (1 mm – 18 cm) occurs in the pancreas in 70% of cases and in the duodenum in 40%.
– VIPoma (6 mm – 20 cm) occurs in the pancreas in 80–90% of cases, and at extrapancreatic sites in 10–20%.
– Glucagonoma (2–40 cm) occurs exclusively in the pancreas.

Imaging Signs

► **Modality of choice**
CT, MRI.

► **Pathognomonic findings**

Often smaller than 3 cm ● Markedly hypervascular ● Larger tumors can exhibit cystic and necrotic changes ● Usually there is no obstruction of the pancreatic duct.

► **CT findings**

Multiphasic thin-slice CT is indicated as some tumors are only detectable in the early arterial phase and others only in the parenchymal or portal venous phase ● Findings include a hypervascular nodule.

► **MRI findings**

Hypointense to surrounding pancreatic tissue on T1-weighted images, hyperintense on T2-weighted images ● Small tumors show homogeneous or ring enhancement ● Larger tumors show heterogeneous enhancement ● *Preferred imaging techniques:* Fat-suppressed T1-weighted SE and GE sequences, T2-weighted FSE and dynamic contrast-enhanced sequences ● Provides diagnostic information comparable with CT.

► **Ultrasound findings**

Round, well demarcated, hypoechoic nodule ● Smooth surface ● Larger tumors show an inhomogeneous echo structure ● Liver metastases are usually readily evaluated ● Small extrapancreatic tumors (gastrinoma) are usually not detected.

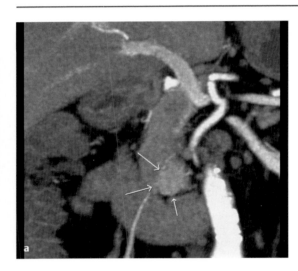

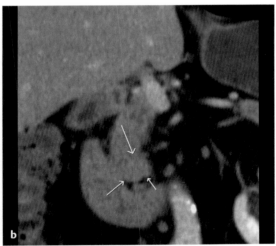

Fig. 3.22 a, b
Benign insulinoma of the head of the pancreas.
a CT, arterial phase. Hypervascular mass (arrows).
b CT, portal venous phase. The mass is now nearly indistinguishable from the surrounding pancreatic parenchyma (arrows).

Fig. 3.23 a, b
Gastrinoma.
a T1-weighted MR image. A small round tumor hypo-intense to the sur-rounding pancreatic parenchyma is visualized at the junction between the body and tail of the pancreas.
b CT. The widened gastric mucosal folds of Zollinger–Ellison syndrome are slightly better visualized. Other findings include a hypervascular gas-trinoma (arrow) in the wall of the stomach measuring a few millimeters in size.

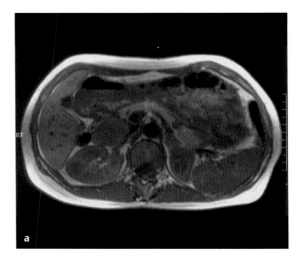

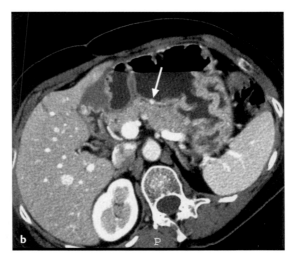

► **Endosonographic findings**
Very sensitive modality for diagnosing multiple small tumors in the pancreas and duodenal or gastric wall ● Combining CT or MRI with endosonography increases diagnostic accuracy to nearly 100%.

► **Interventional techniques**
Angiography with arterial stimulation and venous sampling with selective arterial injection (calcium gluconate to demonstrate insulinomas and secretin to demonstrate gastrinomas) have become less important modalities for locating tumors.

Clinical Aspects

► **Typical presentation**
Symptoms depend on the hormones secreted:
  – *Insulinoma:* Hypoglycemia ● Tachycardia ● Neuropsychiatric symptoms.
  – *Gastrinoma:* Peptic ulcers ● Diarrhea ● Weight loss (Zollinger–Ellison syndrome).
  – *VIPoma:* Watery diarrhea ● Electrolyte imbalance ● Hyperglycemia ● Flush (Verner–Morrison syndrome).
  – *Glucagonoma:* Diabetes ● Diarrhea ● Necrolytic erythema.
  – *Somatostatinoma:* Diabetes mellitus.

► **Therapeutic options**
Treatment involves surgical removal; superficial tumors are only enucleated ● Even patients with metastatic disease benefit from removal of the primary tumor ● Liver metastases can be treated by TACE or TAE.

► **Course and prognosis**
Prognosis is good for benign tumors.

► **What does the clinician want to know?**
Location and number of tumors ● Signs of malignant degeneration.

Differential Diagnosis

Ductal adenocarcinoma	– Hypovascular lesion – Dilatation of the pancreatic duct
Endocrine tumors (not hormonally active)	– Tumors are usually hypovascular or larger – Calcifications in 30% of cases
Solid papillary tumor	– Primarily occurs in young women – Usually cystic areas or hemorrhages
Mucinous cystadenocarcinoma	– Usually more clearly demarcated – Occasionally signs of hemorrhage – Calcifications in the cyst wall – Almost exclusively in women

Tips and Pitfalls

Performing only a single-phase CT and MRI examinations.

Selected Literature

Horton KM et al. Multi-detector row CT of pancreatic islet cell tumors. RadioGraphics 2006; 26: 453–464

Ichikawa T et al. Islet cell tumor of the pancreas: biphasic CT versus MR imaging in tumor detection. Radiology 2000; 216: 163–171

Thoeni RF et al. Detection of small functional islet cell tumors in the pancreas: selection of MR imaging sequences for optimal sensitivity. Radiology 2000; 214: 483–490

Definition

Neuroendocrine tumors of the pancreas whose minimal hormone secretions do not cause specific symptoms.

▶ **Epidemiology**

These account for 30–50% of all neuroendocrine tumors of the pancreas ● Small tumors are occasionally detected incidentally ● Average age at diagnosis is 50–60 years ● No sex predilection.

▶ **Etiology, pathophysiology, pathogenesis**

Hormonally active and nonfunctional tumors can be differentiated by immuno-histochemical examination.

Imaging Signs

▶ **Modality of choice**

CT, MRI.

▶ **Pathognomonic findings**

Often larger than hormonally active tumors (on average larger than 5 cm) ● 80% of tumors are at least partially hypervascular; 20% are hypovascular ● Cystic or necrotic changes are often present ● Larger tumors often exhibit calcifications ● Larger tumors (> 5 cm) are often malignant ● Obstruction of the pancreatic duct may occur with larger tumors and malignant lesions.

▶ **CT findings**

Unenhanced scans demonstrate tumors and calcifications (in 30% of cases) ● The tumors can appear hyperdense, isodense, or hypodense after contrast administration ● Viable components of the tumor enhance with contrast whereas areas of necrosis and cystic degeneration do not.

▶ **MRI findings**

Hypointense or inhomogeneous signal on T1-weighted images ● Signal intensity is increased on T2-weighted images, especially in areas of necrosis and cystic degeneration ● Small tumors show homogeneous or inhomogeneous enhancement ● Larger tumors show heterogeneous contrast enhancement ● *Preferred techniques:* Fat-suppressed T1-weighted SE and GE sequences, T2-weighted FSE and dynamic contrast-enhanced sequences ● Provides diagnostic information comparable with CT.

▶ **Ultrasound findings**

Round, well demarcated hypoechoic nodule ● Small tumors have a smooth surface ● Larger tumors show an inhomogeneous echo structure ● Liver metastases are usually readily evaluated.

▶ **Endosonographic**

Very sensitive modality for detecting small tumors in the pancreas.

Fig. 3.24 a, b Malignant insulinoma. CT. Inhomogeneous tumor of the tail of the pancreas in the arterial (**a**) and portal venous (**b**) phases.

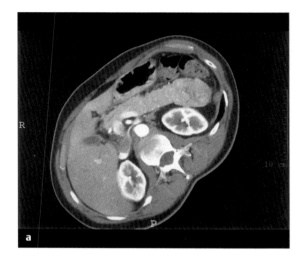

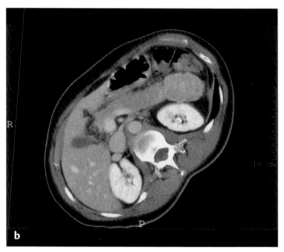

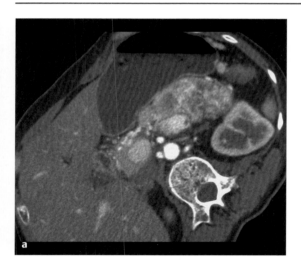

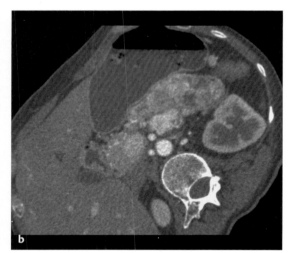

Fig. 3.25 a, b Non-functioning endo-crine tumor of the body and tail of the pancreas in MEN I syndrome. CT. The tumor is markedly inhomogeneous in the arterial phase (**a**) and the portal venous phase (**b**).

Clinical Aspects

▶ **Typical presentation**
Symptoms depend on the size and location of the tumor • Pain • Jaundice • Bowel obstruction • Weight loss • Detection of hormones is not important for the diagnosis.

▶ **Therapeutic options**
Surgical removal.

▶ **Course and prognosis**
Prognosis is good for benign tumors and tumors that have not yet metastasized.

▶ **What does the clinician want to know?**
Location and size of tumors • Signs of malignant degeneration.

Differential Diagnosis

Ductal adenocarcinoma	– Hypovascular lesion
	– Dilatation of the pancreatic duct
Hormonally active endocrine tumors	– Grossly hypervascular
	– Small tumors
	– No calcifications
Solid papillary tumor	– Primarily occurs in young women
	– Usually exhibits cystic components or hemorrhages
Mucinous cystadeno-carcinoma	– Usually more clearly demarcated
	– Occasionally signs of hemorrhage
	– Calcifications in the cyst wall
	– Almost exclusively in women

Tips and Pitfalls

Can be confused with ductal adenocarcinoma.

Selected Literature

Furukawa H et al. Nonfunctioning islet cell tumors of the pancreas: clinical, imaging, and pathologic aspects in 16 patients. Jpn J Clin Oncol 1998; 28: 255–261

Ichikawa T et al. Islet cell tumor of the pancreas: biphasic CT versus MR imaging in tumor detection. Radiology 2000; 216: 163–171

Gouya H et al. CT, endoscopic sonography, and a combined protocol for preoperative evaluation of pancreatic insulinomas. AJR 2003; 181: 987–992

Definition

Malignant, exophytic tumor of the pancreas that does not arise from the ductal system.

► **Epidemiology**
Accounts for 1% of all exocrine tumors of the pancreas ● Average patient age is 50–70 years ● Slightly more common in men.

► **Etiology, pathophysiology, pathogenesis**
Epithelial tumor with acinar differentiation ● Occasionally contains endocrine components (mixed acinar/endocrine carcinoma) ● Tumor can cause hyperlipasemia, leading to necrosis of subcutaneous fatty tissue (painful reddened nodules) and polyarthritis (lytic destruction on radiographs) in 10% of cases ● Shows a slight predilection for the head of the pancreas ● Aggressive tumor that primarily metastasizes to the liver ● Extraabdominal metastases are rare.

Imaging Signs

► **Modality of choice**
CT, MRI.

► **Pathognomonic findings**
Usually large exophytic, well demarcated tumor (2–15 cm in diameter, on average 7–10 cm) ● Lesions less than 5 cm are solid ● Those over 5 cm show necrotic and cystic degeneration ● Hemorrhages may occur ● Calcifications occur in 30% of cases ● Dilation of the bile ducts and pancreatic duct occurs in 20–30% ● Occasionally there is infiltration of the duodenum and stomach ● Vascular infiltration and lymph node metastases are rare.

► **CT and MRI findings**
– *Unenhanced CT and MRI:* Homogeneous or heterogeneous (in cystic degeneration or hemorrhages).
– *CT and MRI after contrast administration:* Solid components enhance homogeneously ● Marked enhancement on CT in the arterial phase ● On MRI, tumor enhances markedly after manganese DPDP administration.

► **Endosonography**
Allows guided biopsy.

Clinical Aspects

► **Typical presentation**
This depends on the location and size of the tumor ● Pressure sensation or pain ● Loss of appetite ● Weight loss ● Nausea ● Obstructive jaundice is rare ● Pancreatic enzymes are occasionally elevated ● Eosinophilia ● AFP is markedly raised.

► **Therapeutic options**
Surgical removal ● Palliative chemotherapy and radiation therapy.

Fig. 3.26 a, b   Acinar cell tumor of the pancreas. CT. Arterial phase (**a**). Large enhancing, partially nodular tumor of the head of the pancreas. Portal venous phase (**b**). Slightly inhomogeneous enhancement, central necrosis. The tumor has been treated with a stent.

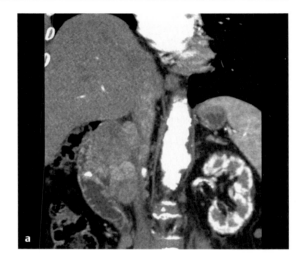

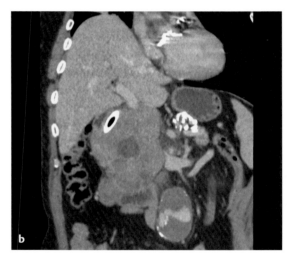

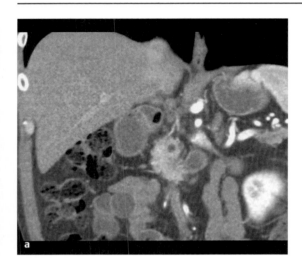

Fig. 3.27 a, b
Acinar cell tumor
of the pancreas. CT.
A relatively small
hypervascular tu-
mor of the head of
the pancreas (**a**)
causing marked
ductal dilation and
parenchymal atro-
phy there, has also
given rise to a large
hypervascular liver
metastasis (**b**).

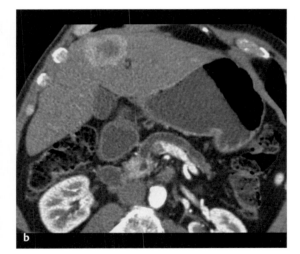

▶ **Course and prognosis**

Prognosis is somewhat better than ductal adenocarcinoma • Prognosis is worse for older patients, lipase-producing tumors, tumors located in the head of the pancreas, and tumors with liver metastases.

▶ **What does the clinician want to know?**

Exclude ductal adenocarcinoma. Size and location of tumor. Metastases in the liver.

Differential Diagnosis

Ductal adenocarcinoma	– Usually smaller lesions – Less enhancement – No calcifications – Infiltrative growth with ill-defined margins
Endocrine tumors *(not hormonally active)*	– Practically indistinguishable – Does not enhance after administration of manganese DPDP
Solid papillary tumor	– Primarily occurs in young women
Mucinous cystadenoma *and cystadenocarcinoma*	– Cysts are better demarcated – Occasionally signs of hemorrhage – Calcifications in the cyst wall – Almost exclusively in women

Tips and Pitfalls

Can be misinterpreted as a ductal adenocarcinoma.

Selected Literature

Klimstra DS et al. Acinar cell carcinoma of the pancreas: a clinicopathologic study of 28 cases. Eur Radiol 2005; 15: 1407–1414

Mustert BR et al. Appearance of acinar cell carcinoma of the pancreas on dual-phase CT. AJR 1998; 171: 1709

Sahani D et al. Functioning acinar cell pancreatic carcinoma: diagnosis on mangafodipir trisodium (Mn-DPDP)-enhanced MRI. J Comput Assist Tomogr 2002; 26: 126–128

Tatli S et al. CT and MRI features of pure acinar cell carcinoma of the pancreas in adults. AJR 2005; 184: 511–519

Definition

Primary or secondary lymphoma of the pancreas.

▶ **Epidemiology**
Primary lymphomas of the pancreas are rare (accounting for less than 2% of extranodal non-Hodgkin lymphomas) and accounts for 1% of all malignant tumors of the pancreas • Average patient age is 50–60 years • Slightly more common in men • Secondary involvement may occur as a result of malignant peripancreatic lymphomas • 30% of cases involve direct infiltration of the pancreas by non-Hodgkin lymphomas.

▶ **Etiology, pathophysiology, pathogenesis**
Incidence is increased in patients with AIDS • These are usually B-cell lymphomas.

Imaging Signs

▶ **Modality of choice**
MRI, CT.

▶ **Pathognomonic findings**
Primary lymphoma: Usually a large tumor (4–14 cm in diameter) • Often occurs in the head of the pancreas • Only peripancreatic lymph nodes are involved • Pancreatic duct is often only displaced or slightly stenosed.
Secondary lymphoma: Continuous spread of lymphomas into the pancreas • Diffuse involvement of the organ.

▶ **MRI findings**
Hypointense or isointense on T1-weighted images, slightly hyperintense on T2-weighted images • Enhances only slightly • Pancreatic duct is displaced or slightly stenosed on MRCP.

▶ **CT findings**
Homogeneously hypodense • Only slight but homogeneous contrast enhancement in circumscribed tumors or generalized involvement (as in pancreatitis).

▶ **Ultrasound findings**
Usually homogeneous • Markedly hypoechoic mass • Surrounded by markedly enlarged lymph nodes.

▶ **Biopsy**
Endoscopic or percutaneous biopsy in primary lymphoma.

▶ **PET findings**
Marked uptake of FDG.

Clinical Aspects

▶ **Typical presentation**
Symptoms are unspecific • Upper abdominal pain (in 70% of cases) • Weight loss (50%) • Jaundice (40%) • Nausea (30%) • Vomiting • Systemic symptoms (fever, night sweats, and weight loss) are present in 10–50% of cases • LDH levels are raised.

Fig. 3.28 a–c Non-Hodgkin lymphoma of the pancreas.
a CT. The image shows a homogeneous mass in the head of the pancreas with part of a plastic stent.
b Unenhanced T1-weighted MR image. Markedly hypointense tumor clearly set off against the rest of the pancreas, which has slightly highly signal intensity.

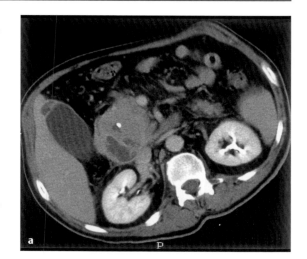

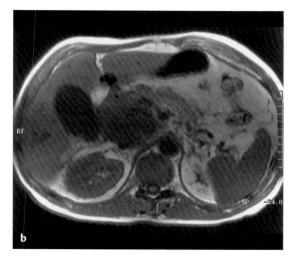

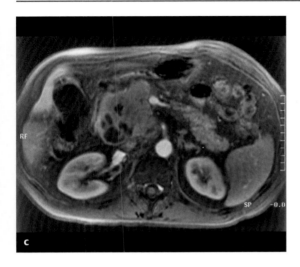

c Tumor in the head of the pancreas shows slight enhancement after contrast administration. The cystic components do not belong to the tumor itself but represent a retention cyst.

▸ **Therapeutic options**
   Combined radiation and chemotherapy ● Role of surgery is controversial.
▸ **Course and prognosis**
   Combined radiation and chemotherapy achieves cure rates approaching 50%.
▸ **What does the clinician want to know?**
   Exclude other tumors or pancreatitis.

Differential Diagnosis

Ductal adenocarcinoma	– More severe obstruction of the pancreatic duct
	– Smaller lymph nodes
	– Liver metastases are common
Pancreatitis	– Peripancreatic fluid collections
	– Elevated amylase and lipase levels

Tips and Pitfalls

Can be misinterpreted as a ductal adenocarcinoma (when a primary lymphoma is suspected, treatment will depend on biopsy findings).

Selected Literature

Cario E et al. Diagnostic dilemma in pancreatic lymphoma. Int J Pancreatol 1997; 22: 67–71

Merkle EM et al. Imaging findings in pancreatic lymphoma. AJR 2000; 174: 671–675

Prayer L et al. CT in pancreatic involvement of non-Hodgkin lymphoma. Acta Radiol 1992; 33: 123–127

Fig. 3.29 a, b
Extensive Burkitt
lymphoma arising
from the retroperi-
toneal region and
infiltrating the pan-
creas. MR image.
Only remnants of
the pancreatic pa-
renchyma are de-
tectable (arrows)
(**a**). After contrast
administration the
lymphoma shows
inhomogeneous en-
hancement (**b**).

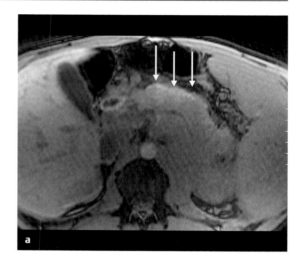

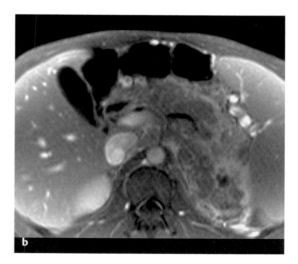

Definition

▶ **Epidemiology**
Rare secondary tumor of the pancreas • Usually occurs only in advanced tumor stages, occasionally long after the initial tumor diagnosis (especially in renal cell carcinoma) • Autopsy studies show an incidence of 3–10%.

▶ **Etiology, pathophysiology, pathogenesis**
Most common primary tumors—renal cell carcinoma, bronchial carcinoma, melanoma, breast carcinoma, colorectal carcinoma, and soft tissue sarcoma.

Imaging Signs

▶ **Modality of choice**
CT, ultrasound.

▶ **Pathognomonic findings**
Usually well-demarcated masses (1.5–2 cm in diameter) • Occasionally multiple lesions are present (20% of cases) • Diffuse infiltration is less common (5%) • Contrast enhancement depends on the primary tumor but is usually heterogeneous • Pancreatic duct and bile duct are dilated (in lesions in the head of the pancreas, 30–40% of cases) • Usually associated with metastases to other organs (50%).

▶ **CT findings**
Hypovascular metastases are readily differentiated from the surrounding parenchyma in the parenchymal phase • Hypervascular metastases (renal cell carcinoma) are usually better visualized in the arterial phase.

▶ **Ultrasound findings**
Usually hypoechoic.

▶ **MRI findings**
Hypointense on T1-weighted images • Metastases from renal cell carcinomas show high signal intensity on T2-weighted images • Marked enhancement occurs after administration of gadolinium • The diagnostic information provided is comparable with CT.

Clinical Aspects

▶ **Typical presentation**
Jaundice (in a metastasis in the head of the pancreas) • Loss of appetite • Weight loss • Pancreatitis occurs less often.

▶ **Therapeutic options**
Depending on the primary tumor, chemotherapy or occasionally resection (in late metastases and isolated metastases of renal cell and breast carcinomas).

▶ **Course and prognosis**
Prognosis is poor • It is most favorable for resection of late metastases of renal cell carcinomas.

Fig. 3.30 a, b
Hypodense metastases of a bronchial carcinoma in the body (**a**) and tail (**b**) of the pancreas. CT.

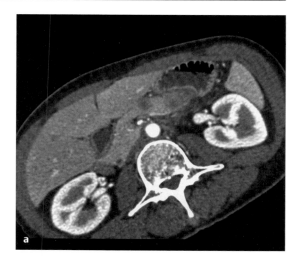

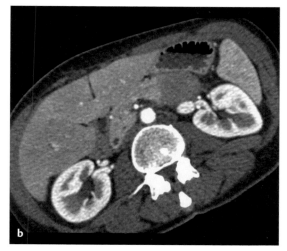

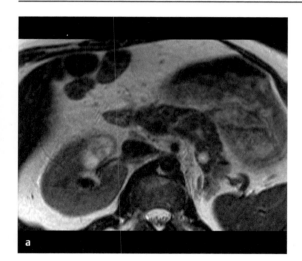

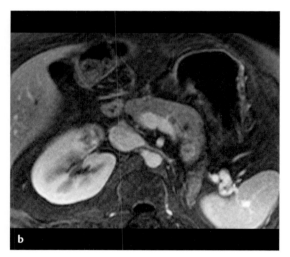

Fig. 3.31 a, b Renal cell carcinoma on the right side.
a T2-weighted MR image. Two hyperintense lesions are visualized, one at the junction of the body and tail of the pancreas and one in the tail itself.
b T1-weighted MR image after contrast administration, the lesion in the tail of the pancreas appears hyperintense whereas the lesion at the junction of the body and tail appears slightly hypointense.

▶ **What does the clinician want to know?**
Evaluate resectability in specific cases • Exclude chronic pancreatitis and other less aggressive tumors.

Differential Diagnosis

Ductal adenocarcinoma	– Usually ill-defined margin
	– Hypovascular lesion
	– Ductal obstruction is practically invariably present
Hormonally active endocrine tumors	– Grossly hypervascular
	– Clinical symptoms
Pancreatic lymphoma	– Usually diffuse involvement of the organ (in diffuse metastatic disease)

Tips and Pitfalls

Can be misinterpreted as a ductal adenocarcinoma.

Selected Literature

Klein KA et al. CT characteristics of metastatic disease of the pancreas. RadioGraphics 1998; 18: 369–378

Merkle EM et al. Metastases to the pancreas. Br J Radiol 1998; 71: 1208–1214

Wernecke K et al. Pancreatic metastases: US evaluation. Radiology 1986; 160: 399–402

Definition

Chronic inflammatory bowel disease with transmural extension.

▶ **Epidemiology**
Usually manifests itself at the age of 15–30 years ● Occurs slightly less frequently in women ● Incidence shows a high degree of regional variation ● There is a slight north–south differential in Europe and the United States.

▶ **Etiology, pathophysiology, pathogenesis**
Disorder involves a genetic disposition with altered immune response to certain pathogens or unknown stimuli ● Inflammation spreads discontinuously from the terminal ileum toward the rectum ● Transmural spread is via fistulas to adjacent bowel loops and through the bowel wall to soft tissue and joints ● Enteric abscesses develop.

Imaging Signs

▶ **Modality of choice**
Endoscopy ● Ultrasound ● MR enteroclysis.

▶ **Pathognomonic findings**
Thickened bowel wall (small bowel > 2 mm, large bowel > 3 mm when distended) ● Marked enhancement in the active phase ● Cobblestone pattern ● Haustra are absent ● Proliferation of fibrotic and fatty tissue (creeping fat sign) ● Normal and affected bowel segments alternate (skip lesions) ● Lymph nodes are enlarged ● *Complications:* Strictures ● Abscesses ● Fistulas.

▶ **Endoscopic findings**
Findings depend on the severity of the disorder ● *Early changes:* Aphthous erosions and ulcerations in healthy mucosa ● *Late changes:* Longitudinal and transverse ulcerations create a cobblestone pattern ● Stenoses ● Fistulas.

▶ **Ultrasound findings**
Important as the primary diagnostic modality ● Thickening of the bowel wall, which in the florid stage is highly perfused (demonstrated by color Doppler or by using ultrasound contrast agents) ● Peristalsis is reduced in the thickened bowel segments ● Stenoses are clearly visualized.

▶ **MRI findings**
The bowel wall is markedly thickened during the active phase ● Pronounced layering may be present ● Bowel wall and inflamed adjacent tissue enhance with contrast ● The acute inflammation (edema) is well visualized on fat-suppressed T2-weighted images ● The bowel wall and surrounding tissue appear hyperintense ● Strictures, fistulas, and abscesses are clearly visualized.

▶ **Findings on enteroclysis**
Mucosal irregularities include ulcerations that in severe cases can create a cobblestone appearance ● Fistulas ● Strictures ● This modality is increasingly being replaced by CT and MRI.

Gastrointestinal Tract (General)

Fig. 4.1 Crohn disease. Image detail from enteroclysis. Normal bowel loops are seen immediately adjacent to inflamed loops showing a cobblestone pattern of longitudinal and transverse ulcerations.

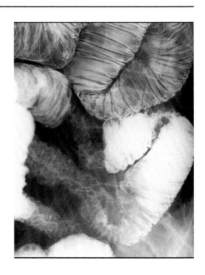

► **CT findings**
In the florid inflammatory phase, the thickened bowel wall enhances markedly with contrast • Complications can be readily evaluated • This modality provides slightly more information than MR enteroclysis • Because it involves relatively high doses of ionizing radiation and patients are generally younger, it should be used with caution.

► **Contrast enema**
Practically no longer used as a diagnostic modality.

► **Findings on plain abdominal radiography**
Can demonstrate toxic megacolon.

► **Capsule endoscopy**
This technique has been successfully employed to visualize discrete changes in the small bowel • Bowel stenosis must be excluded prior to the examination.

Clinical Aspects

► **Typical presentation**
Abdominal pain • Diarrhea • Fever • Weight loss • Signs of malnutrition • Intestinal bleeding when the colon is involved • Anal fistulas.
Extraintestinal manifestations: Arthritis • Iridocyclitis • Aphthous stomatitis • Erythema nodosum • Cholelithiasis • Nephrolithiasis • Primary sclerosing cholangitis • Ankylosing spondylitis.

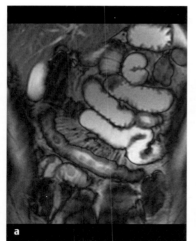

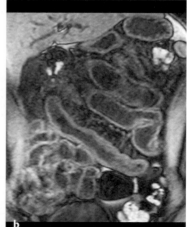

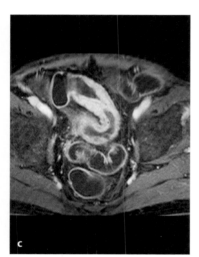

Fig. 4.2 a–c   Crohn disease. MR enteroclysis. The long segment of thickened bowel wall is well visualized on the coronal T2-weighted sequence (**a**) and coronal T1-weighted sequence (**b**). After intravenous contrast administration (**c**), the thickened wall of a terminal ileum loop shows marked enhancement indicative of florid inflammation.

▶ **Therapeutic options**
Prednisone and 5-aminosalicylic acid ● Infliximab ● Surgery for complications such as strictures, fistulas, and abscesses (80% of all patients with Crohn disease undergo surgery at least once during the course of their disease).

▶ **Course and prognosis**
The clinical course can vary considerably ● It is not predictable in any one case ● In the first year there is a high cumulative risk of recurrence of 50% ● Occurrence in the colon increases the risk of colonic carcinoma.

▶ **What does the clinician want to know?**
Exclude other inflammatory or tumorous disorders of the bowel ● Severity ● Activity ● Complications.

Differential Diagnosis

Ulcerative colitis	– Does not involve the small bowel
	– Only the mucosa is affected
	– No fistulas or abscesses
	– Spreads from the rectum to the cecum
Ischemic colitis	– Older patients
	– Vascular changes
	– Reduced perfusion of the bowel wall
Infectious enteritis	– Short medical history
	– Usually there is active peristalsis in the affected segments
Drug-induced damage (NSAIDs)	– Strictures extend only a very short distance
	– Not pronounced in the terminal ileum
Lymphoma	– Wall thickening associated with a dilated lumen (mucosal necrosis)
	– Enlarged mesenteric lymph nodes
Behçet disease	– Indistinguishable

Tips and Pitfalls

Collapsed bowel loops can mimic wall thickening ● MR or CT enteroclysis is not indicated for early and mild forms (only indicated in advanced forms where there is a high probability of complications such as fistula, abscess, or stricture).

Selected Literature

Furakawa A et al. Cross-sectional imaging in Crohn disease. RadioGraphics 2004; 24: 689–702

Sturm EJC et al. Detection of ileocecal Crohn's disease using ultrasound as the primary imaging modality. Eur Radiol 2004; 14: 778–782

Umschaden HW et al. Small bowel disease: Comparison of MR enteroclysis images with conventional enteroclysis and surgical findings. Radiology 2000; 215: 717–725

Definition

Exophytic mesenchymal tumor of the gastrointestinal tract.

▶ **Epidemiology**
   Most common mesenchymal tumor of the gastrointestinal tract • Tumor arise from interstitial cells • Accounts for 3% of all tumors of the gastrointestinal tract • Incidence is 0.7:100 000 • Average patient age is 63 years (ranging from 40 to 70) • Men are affected 1.5 times as often as women • In the setting of Recklinghausen disease, there are multiple tumors confined to the small bowel.

▶ **Etiology, pathophysiology, pathogenesis**
   A kit receptor (CD117) promoting uncontrolled growth and resistance to apoptosis is typically expressed • *Most common locations:* Stomach 50–70%, small bowel 20–35%, colon and rectum 5–7%, esophagus 1–2% • Rarely occurs in the mesentery, omentum, or retroperitoneal region.

Imaging Signs

▶ **Modality of choice**
   CT • Endoscopy in the upper gastrointestinal tract and large bowel.

▶ **Pathognomonic findings**
   Usually a large exophytic tumor measuring 3–10 cm in diameter • No concentric growth in the bowel wall • Aneurysmal dilatation of the bowel lumen is occasionally observed • Calcifications are rare • Lymph node metastases are unusual • No vascular infiltration • Only the size of the tumor indicates its potential for malignancy, not cystic or necrotic degeneration or vascularity • Tumors smaller than 2 cm are usually benign, those over 5 cm are most frequently malignant.

▶ **CT findings**
   Small tumors can enhance markedly • Larger tumors usually enhance heterogeneously • CT can often demonstrate acute bleeding • After treatment with imatinib (Glivec), originally hypervascular tumors acquire a cystic appearance and may exhibit calcifications.

▶ **Endoscopic findings**
   Small tumors can exhibit submucosal growth • Larger tumors penetrate the mucosa and often exhibit ulcerations with increased risk of hemorrhage.

▶ **MRI findings**
   Image quality is often limited by motion artifacts.

▶ **PET findings**
   Appears to be superior in demonstrating early response to imatinib treatment.

Clinical Aspects

▶ **Typical presentation**
   Depends on the location and size of the tumor • Pressure sensation or pain • Bleeding and anemia • Rarely obstructive jaundice and bowel obstruction.

Fig. 4.3 Malignant gastrointestinal stromal tumor. CT. The polypoid tumor is growing into the gastric lumen and has already metastasized to the liver.

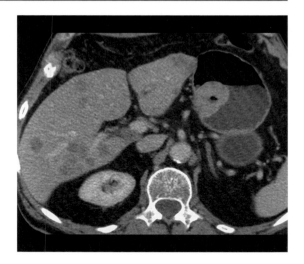

▶ **Therapeutic options**
Surgical removal • Specific molecular treatment with the tyrosine kinase inhibitor imatinib (Glivec) • Radiation therapy and chemotherapy are ineffective.

▶ **Course and prognosis**
At the time of diagnosis 20–30% of tumors are already malignant • 5-year survival rate is 45% • Recurrence after resection is common • Tumors metastasize to the liver and, especially after resection, to the mesentery and omentum.

▶ **What does the clinician want to know?**
Size of tumor and relationship to adjacent structures • Metastases in the liver • Response of tumor and/or metastases to treatment:
– No enhancement in case of moderate decrease in tumor size or unchanged tumor mass (apoptosis instead of necrosis).
– Recurrence or progression: Increase in size, renewed contrast enhancement or enhancing nodules in a tumor of unchanged size, new tumor nodules.

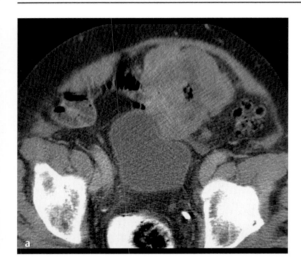

Fig. 4.4 a, b Large gastrointestinal stromal tumor of a small bowel loop in the left lower abdomen. CT. Metastases in the liver and between the liver and diaphragm (**b**).

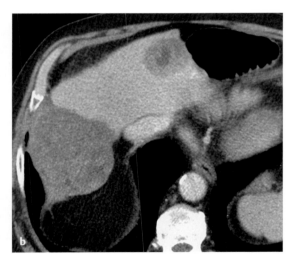

Gastrointestinal Tract (General)

Differential Diagnosis

Adenocarcinoma	– Concentric growth leading to obstruction – Less vascularized than gastrointestinal stromal tumor
Lymphoma	– Usually accompanied by enlarged lymph nodes – Concentric thickening of the bowel wall – Lumen is often dilated
Leiomyosarcoma	– Leads to obstruction – Often metastasizes to the lungs in contrast with gastrointestinal stromal tumors
Carcinoid	– Usually in the distal ileum and appendix – Small hypervascular tumors – Mesenteric tumors often show calcifications and radiating strands into the surrounding fatty tissue

Tips and Pitfalls

Measuring the size of the tumors or metastases is not a suitable criterion of response to treatment • Be alert to the danger of misinterpreting liver metastases as cysts after treatment.

Selected Literature

Burkill GJC et al. Malignant gastrointestinal stromal tumor: distribution, imaging features, and pattern of metastatic spread. Radiology 2003; 226: 527–532

Sandrasegaran K et al. Gastrointestinal stromal tumors: CT and MRI findings. Eur Radiol 2005; 15: 1407–1414

Shankar S et al. Gastrointestinal stromal tumor: new nodule-within-a-mass pattern of recurrence after partial response to imatinib mesylate. Radiology 2005; 235: 892–898

Tran T et al. The epidemiology of malignant gastrointestinal stromal tumors: an analysis of 1458 cases from 1992 to 2000. Am J Gastroenterol 2005; 100: 162–168

Definition

Neuroendocrine tumor of the gastrointestinal tract. The WHO classification (2000) identifies highly differentiated neuroendocrine tumors, highly differentiated neuroendocrine carcinomas, and poorly differentiated neuroendocrine carcinomas. Biologic parameters are also taken into consideration, including location, tumor size, vascular supply, proliferative activity, histology, metastases, invasion of adjacent organs, hormonal activity, and association with clinical syndromes or disorders.

▶ **Epidemiology**
   Accounts for 2% of gastrointestinal tumors • Second most common tumor of the small bowel • Usually occurs between the ages of 40 and 60 years.
▶ **Etiology, pathophysiology, pathogenesis**
   Eighty-five to 90 percent of these tumors arise in the gastrointestinal tract • Most occur in the ileum (25%), appendix (12%), and rectum (14%) • Tumors occur less often in the stomach, duodenum, and pancreas • Tumor growth is slow • 70% are malignant • 30% occur as multifocal lesions • Usually metastasize to liver and bone • Carcinoids secrete serotonin and other mediators.

Imaging Signs

▶ **Modality of choice**
   Multidetector CT, nuclear medicine.
▶ **Pathognomonic findings**
   Small tumors exhibit submucosal growth • Large tumors extend beyond the bowel and infiltrate mesenteric vascular structures • Desmoplastic reaction (stellate pattern of radiating tissue strands in fatty tissue) • Calcifications (in up to 70% of cases) • Small bowel tumors occur as multiple lesions in 30–40%. Metastases in the lymph nodes and liver correlate with tumor size:
   – 20–30% of tumors measuring less than 1 cm produce metastases.
   – 60–80% of tumors measuring 1–2 cm produce lymph node metastases and 20% produce liver metastases.
   – 80% of tumors larger than 2 cm produce lymph node metastases and 40–50% produce liver metastases.
▶ **CT findings**
   Multidetector CT with thin slices shows markedly enhancing submucosal nodules in the early arterial phase (with rapid contrast flow) • This technique is appropriate to demonstrate hypervascular metastases in lymph nodes and liver • Extraintestinal tumor components are visualized as ill-defined masses with calcifications and connective tissue strands radiating in a stellate pattern.
▶ **Somatostatin receptor scintigraphy**
   Suitable modality for detecting a carcinoid or metastases • Sensitivity is 75% as spatial resolution is limited.
▶ **MRI findings**
   Circumscribed nodules • Usually isointense to musculature on T1-weighted images, hyperintense or isointense on T2-weighted images • Occasionally only uniform thickening of the bowel wall is detected • Both forms show marked en-

Fig. 4.5 Multiple carcinoids of the small bowel. Enteroclysis. The carcinoid nodules are identifiable by the round constrictions and the mural defects.

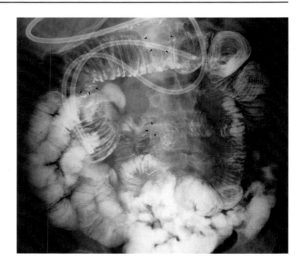

hancement after contrast administration ● Mesenteric tumors appear as stellate masses with radiating strands of tissue ● Liver metastases are hypointense on T1-weighted images and slightly to markedly hyperintense on T2-weighted images (comparable to fluid) ● Tumor appears grossly hypervascular in the early arterial phase ● Large metastases with central necrotic areas show heterogeneous enhancement ● Rarely a centripetal pattern of enhancement like in a hemangioma is observed.

▶ **Findings on enteroclysis**
Submucosal nodules with a smooth surface that project into the lumen of the bowel ● As the tumor expands in size, thickening of the bowel wall and mucosal folds occurs ● Extraintestinal spread of the tumor fixes the adjacent bowel loops and draws them toward the mesentery.

Clinical Aspects

▶ **Typical presentation**
This depends on size and location of the primary tumor and on serotonin secretion ● Clinical manifestation is usually late with extensive local findings and metastases ● The carcinoid syndrome (flush, diarrhea, asthma, and edema) occurs in 10% of patients, usually this is only when liver metastases are present ● Late sequelae include cardiac complications (endocardial fibrosis, pulmonary stenosis, and tricuspid insufficiency) ● Chromogranin A is a suitable tumor marker.

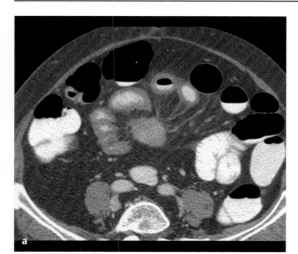

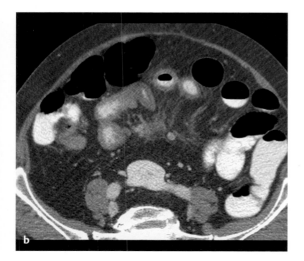

Fig. 4.6 a, b Carcinoid in mesenteric fatty tissue. CT. Tissue radiating in a stellate pattern (**a**) from the carcinoid. Adjacent bowel loops are thickened (**b**).

▶ **Therapeutic options**

Surgical removal of the primary tumor • Radiofrequency ablation or chemoembolization of liver metastases • Somatostatin analogs such as octreotide help alleviate symptoms.

▶ **Course and prognosis**

Five-year survival rate for patients with inoperable primary tumors is 50%; 30% when liver metastases are present • Encasement of mesenteric vascular structures can lead to extensive bowel ischemia • 5-year survival rate is high for patients with tumors in the appendix (> 95%) and rectum (> 85%).

▶ **What does the clinician want to know?**

Metastases in lymph nodes or liver.

Differential Diagnosis

Retractile mesenteritis	– Spread in the mesentery usually patchy
	– No tumor in the small bowel
Lymphomas (non-Hodgkin lymphoma)	– No stellate proliferation of tumor tissue
	– Usually multiple lymphomas
	– No occlusion of mesenteric vascular structures
Gastrointestinal stromal tumor	– In the jejunum and ileum
	– Often large tumor
	– Central necrotic areas
Carcinoma of the small bowel	– Occurs more often in the jejunum
	– Circular growth pattern with obstruction
	– Not as well perfused
Desmoid tumor	– Usually arises from a surgical scar
	– Usually sharply demarcated
	– Patients are younger (20–40 years)

Tips and Pitfalls

Tumor can be misinterpreted as lymph node metastasis.

Selected Literature

Dromain C et al. MR imaging of hepatic metastases caused by neuroendocrine tumors: comparing four techniques. AJR 2003; 180: 121–128

Horton KM et al. Carcinoid tumors of the small bowel: a multitechnique imaging approach. AJR 2004; 182: 559–567

Maccioni F et al. Magnetic resonance imaging of an ileal carcinoid tumor. Correlation with CT and US. Clin Imaging 2003; 27: 403–407

Definition

Acute narrowing or occlusion of mesenteric arteries or veins leading to inadequate blood supply to the bowels.

▶ **Epidemiology**

Incidence is increasing as the population ages ● Of patients presenting with acute abdomen, 1% have mesenteric ischemia.

▶ **Etiology, pathophysiology, pathogenesis**

Two forms: The occlusive form occurs in 75% of cases, with thrombi and emboli in the mesenteric artery and thrombi in the mesenteric vein; 20–30% have the nonocclusive form with hypovolemia ● Many disorders can contribute to re-duced perfusion—bowel obstruction, vasculitis, tumors, medications, radiation therapy ● Over 30% of all patients with acute occlusion of the superior mesen-teric artery have chronic heart disease ● *Sequelae:* These range from reversible functional impairment to transmural bowel necrosis.

Imaging Signs

▶ **Modality of choice**

Multidetector CT with CT angiography ● Angiography.

▶ **Pathognomonic findings**

Complete or partial occlusion of a mesenteric vessel ● Spastic arterial picture (nonocclusive disease) ● Thickening of the bowel wall ● Dilated bowel loops ● (small bowel > 3 cm) ● Mesenteric edema or diffuse intraperitoneal fluid collec-tions ● Reduced perfusion of the thickened bowel wall ● Gas in the bowel wall and in the mesenteric veins.

▶ **Angiographic findings**

The main trunk or a segmental branch of the mesenteric artery is occluded ● In mesenteric venous thrombosis, the mesenteric vein does not fill ● Vascular spasm produces a distinctive vascular picture (angiography remains the superior modality only in this clinical entity).

▶ **Multidetector CT findings**

Lumina of the mesenteric artery and vein are occluded ● Reduced perfusion ● Bowel segments supplied by these vessels are thickened and dilated ● Intramu-ral gas is present ● Perforation or mesenteric fluid is usually readily detectable ● This modality is increasingly becoming the diagnostic gold standard (sensitivity 96%, specificity 94%).

▶ **Ultrasound findings**

Thrombotic occlusion of the mesenteric vein in particular allows rapid diagno-sis ● This is probably also a good modality for diagnosis and follow-up of ische-mic colitis.

▶ **Endoscopic findings**

Indicated in ischemic colitis ● Partial colonoscopy is often sufficient as 85% of all perfusion impairments occur at or below the left colic flexure ● The mucosa may appear edematous, hemorrhagic, or livid with ulcerations.

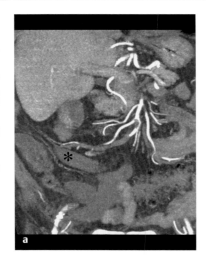 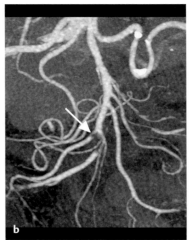

Fig. 4.7 a, b   Acute mesenteric ischemia. Infarction of the terminal ileum (not transmural according to histologic findings). CT.
a   Coronal reconstruction. Thickened terminal ileum loop (asterisk).
b   Embolus in a bifurcation of the superior mesenteric artery (arrow).

▶ **Findings on plain abdominal radiography**
 Findings are often normal in the early phases • Even in more advanced disease, findings are unspecific (picture of paralytic ileus).

Clinical Aspects

▶ **Typical presentation**
 Sudden intense pain (in emboli) or insidious diffuse abdominal pain • Diarrhea occurs shortly thereafter • Abdomen is tender to palpation • Body temperature is slightly elevated • Temporary remission of symptoms is common • This is followed by dramatic worsening of clinical symptoms.
▶ **Therapeutic options**
 Embolectomy or thrombectomy is indicated for proved vascular occlusion • Infarcted bowel loops are resected.
▶ **Course and prognosis**
 Mortality is as high as 60%, and late diagnosis increases the risk • Spontaneous improvement can occur in ischemic colitis.
▶ **What does the clinician want to know?**
 Arterial or venous occlusion.

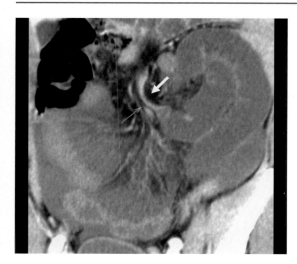

Gastrointestinal Tract (General)

Fig. 4.8 Acute mesenteric ischemia. CT. Bowel loop obstructed by adhesion (large arrow) and obstructed mesenteric vein (small arrow). As a result, the bowel loops on the left are dilated and poorly perfused.

Differential Diagnosis

Chronic inflammatory bowel disease	– Long medical history
	– Normal arterial and venous findings
	– Bowel segments with thickened wall show increased enhancement
	– Stenoses and dilation proximal to the stenoses
Small bowel lymphoma	– Normal arterial and venous findings
	– Thickened wall
	– Lumen is often dilated
	– No perfusion impairments

Tips and Pitfalls

Common errors include waiting too long to perform a multidetector CT examination.

Selected Literature

Kirkpatrick IDC et al. Biphasic CT with mesenteric CT angiography in the evaluation of acute mesenteric ischemia: initial experience. Radiology 2003; 229: 91–98

Ripollés T et al. Sonographic findings in ischemic colitis in 58 patients. AJR 2005; 184: 777–785

Wildermuth S et al. Multislice CT in the pre- and postinterventional evaluation of mesenteric perfusion. Eur Radiol 2005; 15: 1203–1210

Definition

Cystic collections of gas in the subserosal or submucosal layers of the bowel.

► **Epidemiology**
  Usually occurs between the ages of 40 and 70 years • No sex predilection.
► **Etiology, pathophysiology, pathogenesis**
  Primary form (20%): Most often occurs in the colon.
  Secondary form (80%): Most often occurs in the small bowel. Associated with various disorders such as chronic obstructive pulmonary disease (20% of cases) • Occurs after endoscopy (small mucosal tears) • Induced by certain drugs that influence bowel permeability such as steroids and immunosuppressive agents • Caused by autoimmune disorders associated with increased bowel permeability.

Imaging Signs

► **Modality of choice**
  Endoscopy, CT.
► **Pathognomonic findings**
  Polypoid mucosal protrusions • Bubbles or linear streaks of intramural gas.
► **CT findings**
  Primary form: Bubbles of intramural gas without other intestinal pathology • Normal perfusion.
  Secondary form: Bubbles and linear streaks of intramural gas • Dilated bowel loops • Bowel wall is occasionally thickened • Reduced perfusion • Occasionally findings include gas in the mesenteric veins and portal vein or free intraabdominal gas.
► **Findings on plain abdominal radiography**
  Round or linear radiolucencies along the wall of the bowel.
► **Findings on double contrast studies**
  Polypoid filling defects create a grotesque mucosal surface.
► **Endoscopic findings**
  Flat, firm but elastic, projections that can be impressed; the overlying mucosa appears normal.

Clinical Aspects

► **Typical presentation**
  Usually an incidental finding at endoscopy, on radiographs, or during surgery • Diarrhea • Mucus discharge • Bleeding • Constipation. Complications (in 3% of cases): Volvulus • Obstruction • Bleeding • Perforation.
  In secondary pneumatosis, complications depend on the associated disease • In necrosis of the bowel, they include acute abdomen.
► **Therapeutic options**
  This depends on the underlying disorder • Primary forms usually do not require treatment • In ischemia, resection of the necrotic bowel is indicated.

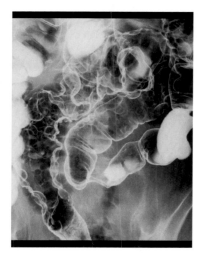

Fig. 4.9 Primary form of pneumatosis intestinalis. Double contrast study of the colon. Severe idiopathic pneumatosis in the sigmoid colon with irregular wall contours and cushion-like polypoid mucosal surface.

▶ **Course and prognosis**
   This depends on the underlying disorder.
▶ **What does the clinician want to know?**
   Necrosis of the bowel or harmless form?

Differential Diagnosis

Ischemia	– Occlusion of the mesenteric artery or one of its branches
	– Decreased perfusion of the wall of the bowel after contrast administration
	– Fluid in the mesentery
Polyposis	– Isodense to soft tissue on CT
	– On double contrast technique they appear sessile or pedunculated

Tips and Pitfalls

Primary form can be misinterpreted as bowel ischemia.

Selected Literature

Boerner RM et al. Pneumatosis intestinalis. Two case reports and a retrospective review of the literature from 1985 to 1995. Dig Dis Sci 1996; 41: 2272–2285
Kernagis LY et al. Pneumatosis intestinalis in patients with ischemia: correlation of CT findings and prognosis. Radiology 2003; 180: 733–736
Pear BL et al. Pneumatosis intestinalis: a review. Radiology 1998; 207: 13–19

Fig. 4.10 a, b Pneumatosis in the ascending colon with free fluid around the pole of the cecum (**a**). This was attributable to ischemic damage from an obstructive tumor at the junction of the descending colon and sigmoid colon (arrow in **b**).

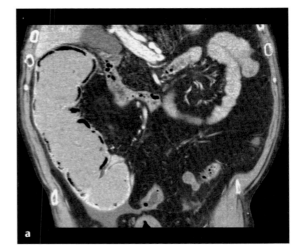

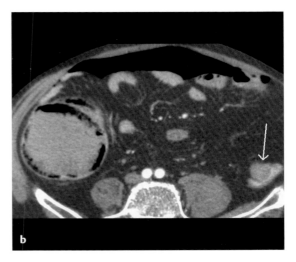

Definition

▶ **Epidemiology**
   Half of all cases occur in patients over 60 years ● Men are affected more often
   than women ● About 1 in 4 cases of acute bleeding is life threatening ● Occult
   bleeding occurs in 1–2% of the asymptomatic population over 40 years of age.

▶ **Etiology, pathophysiology, pathogenesis**
   A distinction is made between bleeding in the upper and lower gastrointestinal
   tract—the source of the bleeding is either proximal to the duodenojejunal flexure
   (80–90%) or distal to it (10–20%) ● *Severity of bleeding:* Acute or occult bleeding ● Common causes of hematemesis and melena are gastroduodenal ulcers
   (> 50%), esophageal varices (15%), Mallory–Weiss syndrome (5%), and tumors
   (5%) ● Common causes of hematochezia (acute blood in the stool) are colonic diverticulum (40%), angiodysplasia (25%), polyps, colorectal carcinoma (15%), ulcerative colitis (10%), hemorrhoids, and fissures.

Imaging Signs

▶ **Modality of choice**
   Endoscopy ● Multidetector CT ● Angiography.

▶ **Pathognomonic findings**
   Leakage of contrast agent from a blood vessel (direct sign) ● Abrupt termination
   of a vascular structure ● Vascular changes such as pseudoaneurysms ● Tumor
   (e.g., gastrointestinal stromal tumor) ● Thickening of the bowel wall with increased perfusion.

▶ **Endoscopic findings**
   Directly demonstrates bleeding ● Endoscopy also has the capability of achieving
   hemostasis.

▶ **CT findings**
   Extravasation of contrast agent into the intestinal lumen ● Reconstruction techniques can visualize findings similarly to angiography, thus demonstrating vessel alterations responsible for hemorrhage ● This study is usually indicated
   when endoscopy fails to demonstrate the cause of the bleeding.

▶ **Angiographic findings**
   Directly visualizes extravasation of contrast agent ● Demonstrates vascular
   changes indicative of imminent bleeding ● Angiography is particularly indicated
   when interventional hemostasis is aimed at.

▶ **Findings on capsule endoscopy**
   Increasingly used with great success in detecting occult bleeding.

▶ **Enteroclysis**
   Has a secondary role ● Provides very little diagnostic information ●

▶ **Nuclear medicine**
   Nuclear medicine imaging methods (using ^{99}Tc-labeled erythrocytes) ● Used in
   hemodynamically stable patients or in the presence of occult bleeding.

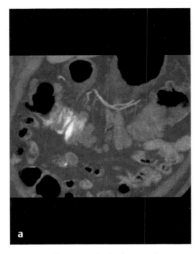
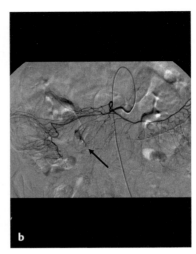

Fig. 4.11 a, b Diverticular hemorrhage.
a CT. Acute leakage of contrast agent into the lumen of the transverse colon.
b Angiography showing leakage of contrast material (arrow).

Clinical Aspects

▸ **Typical presentation**
Acute hemorrhage: Hematemesis ● Melena ● Hematochezia ● Sweats ● Hypotension ● Shock.
Chronic hemorrhage: Recurrent bleeding ● Anemia.

▸ **Therapeutic options**
Endoscopic hemostasis ● Transarterial hemostasis (clinical success rate is over 80%, better for bleeding in the lower gastrointestinal tract than in the upper tract).

▸ **Course and prognosis**
Bleeding in the lower gastrointestinal tract is not usually acutely life threatening and stops spontaneously in 80–95% of cases ● Bleeding from the upper gastrointestinal tract tends to recur, usually within 3 days ● With recurrent bleeding, the mortality increases by a factor of 5–10.

▸ **What does the clinician want to know?**
Location of the hemorrhage ● Cause of bleeding.

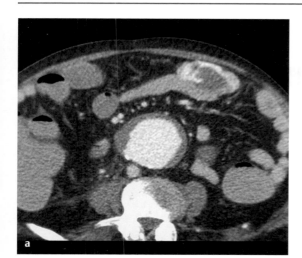

Fig. 4.12 a, b Acute leakage of contrast agent into a loop of the ileum (**a**) in a patient with multiple aneurysms of the mesenteric vessels and hepatic artery (arrows in **b**).

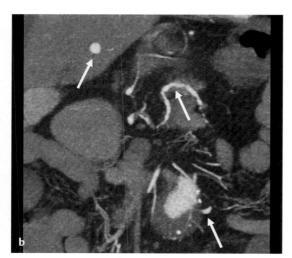

Differential Diagnosis

Esophageal varices	– Cirrhosis of the liver or portal vein occlusion
	– Varices in the wall of the stomach and esophagus
Angiodysplasia	– Large arterial feeder occasionally present
	– Nodular to patchy pattern of increased enhancement in the intestinal mucosa
	– Very early and intense filling of the associated veins
Diverticular hemorrhage	– Diverticulosis
	– Extravasation of contrast agent from the diverticula
Bleeding from a tumor	– Exophytic or intramural tumor (e.g., gastrointestinal stromal tumor)
Vascular malformations	– Pseudoaneurysms or ectatic vessels
Meckel Diverticulum	– Angiography demonstrates vitelline artery
	– Enteroclysis or CT demonstrates an outpouching, usually 50–60 cm from the ileocecal valve

Tips and Pitfalls

Errors include delayed use of radiologic imaging modalities in bleeding from unknown sources and bleeding from known sources that cannot be sufficiently controlled endoscopically.

Selected Literature

Ernst O et al. Helical CT in acute lower gastrointestinal bleeding. Eur Radiol 2003; 13: 114–117

Ko HS et al. Blutungslokalisation mittels 4-Zeilen-Spiral-CT bei Patienten mit klinischen Zeichen einer akuten gastrointestinalen Hämorrhagie. Fortschr Röntgenstr 2005; 177: 1649–1654

Tew K et al. MDCT of acute lower gastrointestinal bleeding. AJR 2004; 182: 427–430

Definition

Saccular dilations or diverticulumlike outpouchings of the visceral vessels.

▶ **Epidemiology**

Aneurysms of the splenic and hepatic arteries are the most common abdominal lesions and together account for 80% of all visceral aneurysms.

▶ **Etiology, pathophysiology, pathogenesis**

Arteriosclerosis ● Amyloidosis ● Infection ● Trauma ● Surgery ● Radiologic intervention ● Arteritis ● Pseudoaneurysms in the setting of chronic pancreatitis are a special case. These lesions arise due to enzymatic digestion of a vascular structure or erosion of a pseudocyst into a vascular structure (splenic, pancreaticoduodenal or gastroduodenal artery).

Imaging Signs

▶ **Modality of choice**

Multidetector CT, angiography.

▶ **Pathognomonic findings**

Saccular dilations in vascular segments (usually genuine aneurysms) ● Circumscribed outpouchings (usually pseudoaneurysms) ● Thromboses or calcifications are occasionally detected ● Signs of hemorrhage are seen in parenchymal organs (especially the liver), in pancreatic pseudocysts, and in the gastrointestinal tract.

▶ **Multidetector CT findings**

MIP reconstructions from images obtained in the arterial phase visualize vascular structures and complications with precision comparable to angiography ● Usually CT provides sufficient information to determine whether radiologic intervention is indicated.

▶ **Angiographic findings**

Visualizes vascular structures with slightly greater detail. However, this is an invasive technique that is no longer indicated where multidetector CT is available ● Indicated when an interventional procedure is required.

▶ **Ultrasound findings**

Aneurysms and pseudoaneurysms of the hepatic artery and pseudoaneurysms in chronic pancreatitis are readily detectable.

▶ **MRI findings**

MR angiography provides diagnostic information of a quality similar to CT angiography but is a considerably more elaborate examination.

Fig. 4.13 a, b
Visceral aneurysms.
CT. Axial (**a**) and
coronal (**b**) MIP re-
constructions. Se-
vere aneurysms of
the celiac trunk and
common hepatic
artery.

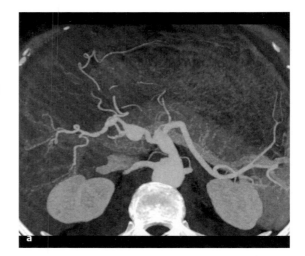

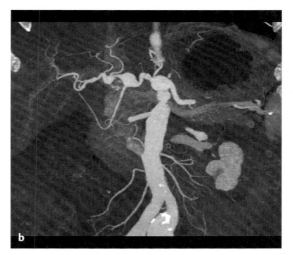

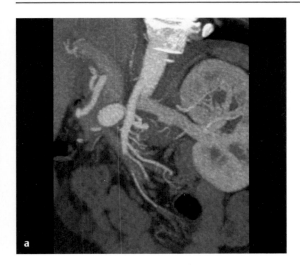

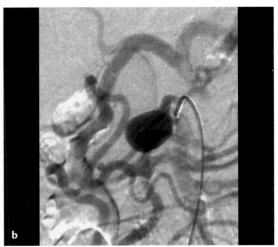

Fig. 4.14 a, b
Aneurysm of the
superior mesenteric
artery.
a CT. The affected
vessel is readily
identified.
b Angiography.
Aneurysm with a
short neck that
is accessible for
embolization with
coils.

Clinical Aspects
. . . .

▶ **Typical presentation**
  Aneurysms are occasionally an incidental finding with modern imaging modalities • Spontaneous rupture leads to acute abdomen • Unspecific abdominal symptoms can precede the acute event for months.

▶ **Therapeutic options**
  Embolization • Surgical ligation.

▶ **Course and prognosis**
  This depends on the underlying disorder and the specific vessel • Spontaneous rupture with a high rate of mortality (> 30 %) occurs in 3–10 % of all patients with aneurysms of the splenic artery.

▶ **What does the clinician want to know?**
  Presence of pseudoaneurysms or aneurysms larger than 2 cm (increased risk) • Is radiologic intervention feasible?

Tips and Pitfalls
. . . .

Obtaining multidetector CT images in an inadequate phase and with insufficient flow of the contrast agent.

Selected Literature

Berceli SA. Hepatic and splenic artery aneurysms. Semin Vasc Surg 2005; 18: 196–201

Iannaccone R et al. Multislice CT angiography of mesenteric vessels. Abdom Imaging 2004; 29: 146–152

Soudack M et al. Celiac artery aneurysm: diagnosis by color Doppler sonography and three-dimensional CT angiography. J Clin Ultrasound 1999; 27: 49–51

Definition

▶ **Epidemiology**
Zenker diverticula are demonstrated in 1% of all contrast studies of the esophagus.

▶ **Etiology, pathophysiology, pathogenesis**
Seventy percent occur at the level of Killian's triangle (cervical or Zenker diverticulum) • 22% occur at the level of the tracheal bifurcation (traction diverticulum) • 8% occur just above the diaphragm (epiphrenic diverticulum).
Zenkel diverticula arise at a weak point between the oblique and transverse fibers of the inferior pharyngeal constrictor • The cause seems to be incomplete relaxation of the upper esophageal sphincter • Traction diverticula are usually caused by inflamed lymph nodes in tuberculosis and histoplasmosis • Epiphrenic diverticula can be associated with motility disturbances • Rare form—intramural pseudodiverticula resulting from dilated submuscular glands and presenting as multiple fistula-like outpouchings.

Imaging Signs

▶ **Modality of choice**
Barium swallow.

▶ **Pathognomonic findings**
Contrast-filled outpouching of the esophagus • Usually located on the left posterior aspect of the upper esophagus (Zenker diverticulum) • Prominent cricopharyngeus muscle (Zenker diverticulum) • Hairline fistula-like channels through the wall of the esophagus (intramural pseudodiverticula).

▶ **Barium swallow**
Zenker diverticulum: Contrast-filled outpouching below the hypopharynx • Lateral images show a posterior evagination, which in larger diverticula can extend inferiorly into the mediastinum • The neck of the diverticulum is visible above the constriction of the esophagus by the cricopharyngeus muscle • Contrast agent remains in the diverticulum and can empty into the hypopharynx when the patient swallows again.
Traction diverticulum: Usually a small linear or triangular outpouching • Diverticulum empties when the esophagus collapses.
Epiphrenic diverticulum: Contrast-filled outpouching, usually occurring on the right side • Often associated with hiatal hernia or achalasia.

▶ **CT findings**
In traction diverticula, it is often possible to visualize the relationship between the diverticulum and enlarged or calcified lymph nodes.

▶ **Endoscopic findings**
Often an incidental finding • Usually the neck of the diverticulum is well visualized • Intramural pseudodiverticulum presents with a typical picture.

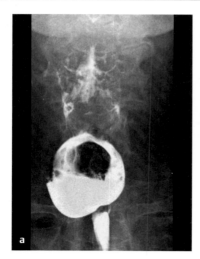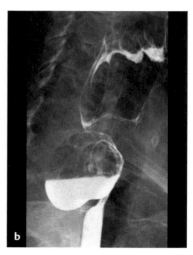

Fig. 5.1 a, b   Large Zenker diverticulum. Conventional A-P (**a**) and lateral (**b**) radiographs after oral contrast administration (barium swallow). The lateral film shows constriction at the level of the cricopharyngeus muscle.

Clinical Aspects

▸ **Typical presentation**
  Regurgitation of undigested food and saliva ● Halitosis ● Occasionally dysphagia.
▸ **Therapeutic options**
  Only symptomatic Zenker diverticula require treatment ● Small diverticula are treated by endoscopic diverticulectomy ● When this is not feasible, treatment includes surgical removal.
▸ **Course and prognosis**
  Usually uncomplicated ● Failure to exercise proper care in performing endoscopy or placing a gastric tube can lead to iatrogenic perforation of diverticula.
▸ **What does the clinician want to know?**
  Size and location of the diverticulum.

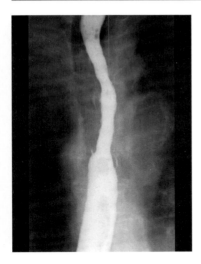

Fig. 5.2 Conventional radiograph after oral contrast administration (barium swallow). A large segment of the upper third of the esophagus shows slight constriction with small intramural diverticula.

Differential Diagnosis

Oropharyngeal pouch (DD to Zenker diverticulum)	– Transient outpouching of the thyrohyoid membrane resembling a pharyngocele – Smaller than a Zenker diverticulum – Does not extend past the posterior margin of the esophagus
Perforation (DD to traction diverticula and pseudo-diverticula)	– Pain and fever – Pneumomediastinum – Does not empty when the esophagus collapses
Hiatal hernia (DD to epiphrenic diverticulum)	– Head-dependent positioning and pressing demonstrate a relationship to the stomach – Gastric folds in the herniated tissue

Tips and Pitfalls

Lesion can be misinterpreted as a perforation (especially in a traction diverticulum).

Selected Literature

Canon CL et al. Intramural tracking: a feature of esophageal intramural pseudodiverticulosis. AJR 2000; 175: 371–374

Fasano NC et al. Epiphrenic diverticulum: clinical and radiographic findings in 27 patients. Dysphagia 2003; 18: 9–15

Ponette E et al. Radiological aspects of Zenker's diverticulum. Hepatogastroenterology 1992; 39: 115–122

Definition

▶ **Epidemiology**

Most common malignant tumor of the esophagus • Accounts for 1% of all carcinomas and 7% of all gastrointestinal carcinomas • Prevalence is 3 : 100 000 • Incidence of the tumor has increased in the past 20 years, and its typical location and histologic findings have also changed—the distally proliferating adenocarcinoma has become more common than the squamous cell carcinoma • It is considerably more common in men (by a ratio of 5 : 1) • Most often occurs between the ages of 40 and 60 years • 25% occur in the upper third of the esophagus, 50% in the middle third, and 25% in the lower third.

▶ **Etiology, pathophysiology, pathogenesis**

Squamous cell carcinoma (50–70% of cases): Most important risk factors are alcohol misuse and smoking • Ingestion of toxic substances in food (aflatoxins and nitrosamines) • Caustic injury due to alkali • Achalasia • Barrett esophagus • Scleroderma.

Adenocarcinoma (30–50% of lesions): Risk factors: Gastroesophageal reflux, Barrett esophagus.

Imaging Signs

▶ **Modality of choice**

Endoscopy • Endosonography • Barium swallow • CT.

▶ **Pathognomonic findings**

Narrowing of the lumen • Rigid irregular contour • Polypoid contours are occasionally observed • Thickened wall and early spread into the mediastinum • Enlarged lymph nodes.

▶ **Barium swallow**

Irregular contour and narrowing of the lumen • The degree of stenosis and length can be reliably determined • Indicated especially in high-grade stenosis when the tumor does not allow the passage of an endoscope.

▶ **Endoscopy and endosonography**

Determination of the length and extent of the tumor • Guiding a biopsy • T and N classification with endosonography is relatively reliable.

▶ **CT findings**

Esophageal wall is thickened and enhances only slightly with contrast • Oral contrast administration improves visualization of the stenosis.

  – *Stage I:* Circumscribed tumor with slight thickening of the wall (3–5 mm).
  – *Stage II:* Circumscribed thickening of the wall (> 5 mm), smooth external contour.
  – *Stage III:* Spread to mediastinal structures such as lymph nodes, tracheobronchial tree, pericardium, and aorta.
  – *Stage IV:* Involvement of subdiaphragmatic lymph nodes, metastases to lung and pleura, liver, and adrenal glands.

▶ **MRI findings**

Diagnostic value is limited due to motion artifacts.

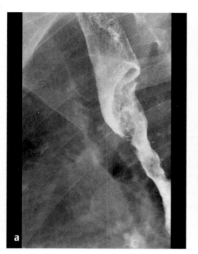

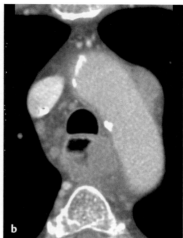

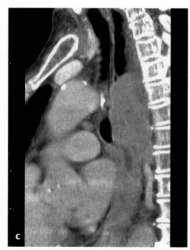

Fig. 5.3 a–c Large esophageal carcinoma in the upper to middle third.
a Double contrast image. Esophageal constriction with irregular contour.
b CT. Eccentrically growing esophageal carcinoma.
c CT, sagittal view. Extensive tumor infiltration in the prevertebral segment.

Fig. 5.4 a, b
Esophageal carcinoma on CT. Exophytic intraluminal tumor of the distal esophagus (arrows) that ends at the cardia.

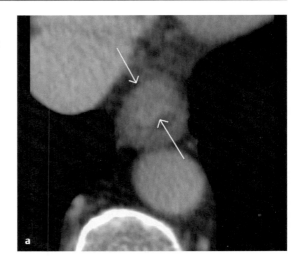

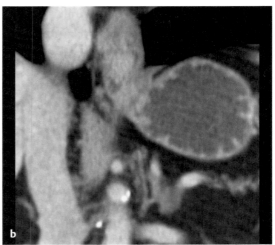

▶ **PET findings**
FDG-PET is superior for demonstrating regional and distant metastases ● Diagnostic precision in demonstrating tumors varies with the stage of the tumor (40 % for T1 to 100 % for T4) ● Can be used effectively with CT, a combination that could become an important modality in staging.

Clinical Aspects

▶ **Typical presentation**
Increasing dysphagia, initially with solid food and later with low-residue foods and liquids as well ● Retrosternal pain and burning sensation ● Regurgitation ● Singultus.

▶ **Therapeutic options**
Resection of the tumor with removal of the mediastinal, pericardial, and superior pancreatic lymph nodes (complete resection is possible in 40 %) ● Patients with inoperable tumors are treated with radiation therapy and chemotherapy ● In advanced cases, endoscopic palliative treatment includes laser therapy and stent implantation.

▶ **Course and prognosis**
This depends on the location and extent of the tumor and on the number of involved lymph nodes ● Mean 5-year survival rate is less than 10 % ● Only 10 % of all lesions are early carcinomas with a chance of cure.

▶ **What does the clinician want to know?**
Location and length ● N and M classification.

Differential Diagnosis

Inflammatory stricture	– Gradually turns into a stenosis
	– Often still contributes to peristalsis
	– Inner contour is smooth or only slightly irregular
	– History of chronic reflux or caustic injury
Submucosal tumor	– Polypoid projection into the lumen
	– Smooth mucosal contour

Tips and Pitfalls

Lesion can be misinterpreted as a benign stricture.

Selected Literature

Gupta S et al. Usefulness of barium studies for differentiating benign and malignant strictures of the esophagus. AJR 2003; 180: 737–744

Iyer BB et al. Diagnosis, staging, and follow-up of esophageal cancer. AJR 2003; 181: 785–793

Kato H et al. The incremental effect of positron emission tomography on diagnostic accuracy in the initial staging of esophageal carcinoma. Cancer 2005; 103: 148–156

Definition

Partial or complete herniation of the stomach into the thorax • Mixed forms of axial and paraesophageal hernias are common.

- *Axial hernia* (sliding hiatal hernia, > 90 % of cases): Axial herniation of the cardia into the thorax.
- *Paraesophageal hernia* (< 5 %): Cardia remains in its normal position • Part of the stomach (usually the fundus) herniates into the thorax.
- *Most severe form:* Herniation of the entire stomach into the thorax ("upside down stomach").

▶ **Epidemiology**
Prevalence increases with age • Over 50 % of people over 60 years have axial hernias • Occurs more often in women.

▶ **Etiology, pathophysiology, pathogenesis**
Increased intraabdominal pressure (obesity and pregnancy) • Defects in the esophageal hiatus (congenital or traumatic) • Weakness in the phrenoesophageal membrane.

Imaging Signs

▶ **Modality of choice**
Endoscopy, barium swallow.

▶ **Pathognomonic findings**
Gastric mucosa in the thorax (axial hernia) • Portions of the stomach are adjacent to the distal esophagus • Irregular distal esophageal mucosa due to reflux.

▶ **Endoscopic findings**
Cardia lies superior to the diaphragm • When the gastroscope is inverted, the opening of the paraesophageal hernia is detectable • Gastroesophageal reflux is best evaluated with this modality.

▶ **Findings on barium swallow**
Axial hernia: Longitudinal gastric folds above the level of the diaphragm.
Paraesophageal hernia: Chest images show a cavity with or without a fluid level adjacent or posterior to the esophagus • The extent and reversibility of a paraesophageal hernia is best evaluated with a barium swallow • Double-contrast studies show inflammatory and ulcerative mucosal changes.

▶ **CT findings**
Frequent incidental finding on CT of the chest and abdomen • Diaphragmatic dehiscence (> 15 mm) • Occasionally the herniated tissue in a paraesophageal hernia also include portions of the omentum • A collapsed, herniated portion of the stomach can mimic a mass in the lower esophagus • An "upside down stomach" is best visualized on thin slices with a reconstruction technique.

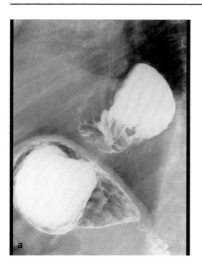

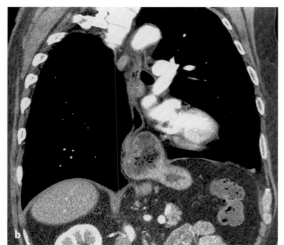

Fig. 5.5 a, b   Hiatal hernia.
a Upper gastrointestinal series on lateral film. The gastric fundus has herniated into the thorax.
b CT, coronal reconstruction. The cardia and fundus have herniated into the thorax.

Fig. 5.6 a, b   Upside down stomach.
a Upper gastrointestinal series. Entire stomach has herniated into the thorax.
b Axial CT. Entire stomach has herniated into the thorax. The pancreas (asterisk) is also displaced into the thorax.

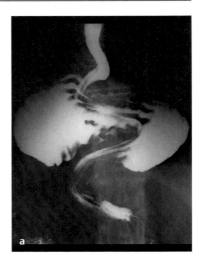

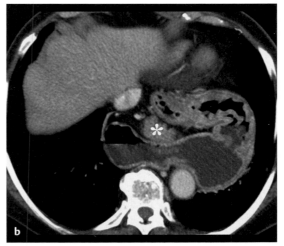

Clinical Aspects

▶ **Typical presentation**
Axial sliding hernias are often an incidental finding and are usually asymptomatic • Associated with gastroesophageal reflux in less than 50% of cases • Paraesophageal hernias are associated with retrosternal pressure sensation, eructation, and dysphagia • Reflux symptoms are not usually present • Complications of paraesophageal hernias may include ulcerations and chronic bleeding • Severe complications such as obstruction, strangulation, and perforation are rare.

▶ **Therapeutic options**
There is no treatment for axial sliding hernia apart from management of the gastroesophageal reflux • Surgical correction is indicated for paraesophageal hernia.

▶ **Course and prognosis**
In paraesophageal hernia, surgery is indicated even in asymptomatic cases due to the risk of complications.

▶ **What does the clinician want to know?**
Exclude an abscess (on the thoracic image) • Does the condition require treatment?

Differential Diagnosis

Epiphrenic diverticulum	– Saccular outpouching of the distal esophagus
	– Arises from the lateral wall of the esophagus

Tips and Pitfalls

Paraesophageal hernia can be misinterpreted as an abscess.

Selected Literature

Chen YM et al. Multiphasic examination of the esophagogastric region for strictures, rings, and hiatal hernia: Evaluation of the individual techniques. Gastrointest Radiol 1985; 10: 311–316

Insko EK et al. Benign and malignant lesions of the stomach: evaluation of CT criteria for differentiation. Radiology 2003; 228: 166–171

Pupols A et al. Hiatal hernia causing a cardia pseudomass on computed tomography. J Comput Assist Tomogr 1984; 8: 699–700

Definition

▶ **Epidemiology**
Most common malignant tumor of the stomach • Incidence has been decreasing for years (25:100 000 in men, 9:100 000 in women) • Distal gastric carcinomas are decreasing, tumors close to the cardia are increasing • Peak incidence is after age 50 years.

▶ **Etiology, pathophysiology, pathogenesis**
Risk factors: *Helicobacter pylori* infection • Drinking water containing nitrates • Smoked foods • Type A gastritis • Ménétrier disease • Risk is two to three greater in immediate relatives • 90% of all carcinomas are adenocarcinomas.

Imaging Signs

▶ **Modality of choice**
Endoscopy • Endosonography • CT.

▶ **Pathognomonic findings**
Lumen is narrowed • Relief of the longitudinal folds is interrupted • Rigid, irregular contour • Polypoid contours are occasionally observed • Wall is thickened (> 1 cm) • Enlarged lymph nodes.

▶ **Endoscopy and endosonographic findings**
Determining the length and extent of the tumor and guiding a biopsy • T and N classification with endosonography is relatively reliable.

▶ **CT findings**
Thickened gastric wall that only enhances slightly with contrast • The thickened wall appears better demarcated after oral administration of water • Wall thickening is partially eccentric, partially concentric • Occasionally there is a bizarre internal contour • Infiltration of surrounding fatty tissue appears as radiating strands of tumor tissue • The extent of tumor in the serosa is especially well demonstrated on thin-slice images on multidetector CT (diagnostic precision > 90%) • This modality also greatly facilitates evaluation of liver metastases and lymph node involvement.

▶ **Findings on upper gastrointestinal series**
Irregular contour and narrowing of the lumen • Severity of stenosis and length can be accurately determined • Now only used as a supplementary modality.

▶ **MRI findings**
Circumscribed asymmetrical thickening of the wall, which enhances either more or less than the surrounding gastric wall.

Clinical Aspects

▶ **Typical presentation**
Uncharacteristic upper abdominal pain (ulcer pain) • Fatigue • Weight loss • Anemia • Hematemesis.

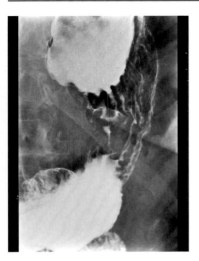

Fig. 6.1 Gastric carcinoma. Upper gastrointestinal series. A mass with a central necrosis is visualized in the middle of the stomach along the lesser curvature, where it disrupts the gastric folds.

▶ **Therapeutic options**
The mucosa may be resected endoscopically in certain forms of early carcinoma • Local tumors are treated by total or subtotal gastrectomy • In inoperable local tumors, treatment aims to control complications such as obstruction and bleeding • Chemotherapy.

▶ **Course and prognosis**
In early carcinomas, the 5-year survival rate is 85–100% • In advanced tumors it is 0–35%.

▶ **What does the clinician want to know?**
Location and extent • N and M staging.

Differential Diagnosis

Gastritis	– Relatively uniform thickening of the gastric folds
	– Relatively uniform thickening of the gastric wall
	– Contributes to peristalsis
Gastric lymphoma	– Significantly thickened gastric wall
	– Thickened folds
Gastrointestinal stromal tumor	– Large exophytic mass
	– Often with extensive extraintestinal component
Ménétrièr disease	– Uniformly thickened folds

Fig. 6.2 a, b Gastric carcinoma. Unenhanced T1-weighted MR image. Circular thickening of the wall of the antrum.

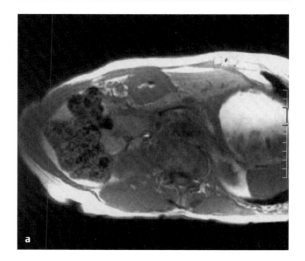

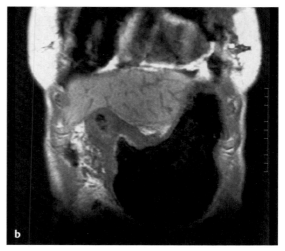

Stomach and Duodenum

Tips and Pitfalls

Overstaging and understaging.

Selected Literature

Habermann CR et al. Preoperative staging of gastric adenocarcinoma: comparison of helical CT and endoscopic ultrasound. Radiology 2004; 230: 465–471

Insko EK et al. Benign and malignant lesions of the stomach: evaluation of CT criteria for differentiation. Radiology 2003; 228: 166–171

Kumano S et al. T staging of gastric cancer: role of multi-detector row CT. Radiology 2005; 237: 961–966

Definition

Herniation of mucosa and muscularis mucosa through the duodenal wall.

▶ **Epidemiology**
Prevalence according to ERCP findings is 25% ● Increases with age ● Slightly more common in women ● Usually an incidental finding at endoscopy or on cross-sectional imaging studies.

▶ **Etiology, pathophysiology, pathogenesis**
Seventy-five percent of all diverticula occur in the immediate vicinity of the papilla (juxtapapillary diverticula) ● Often associated with bile duct stones ● *Complications:* Ectopic bacterial colonization and enteroliths.

Imaging Signs

▶ **Modality of choice**
CT, MRCP.

▶ **Pathognomonic findings**
Air or fluid-filled outpouching of the duodenum ● Occurs on the medial side of the duodenum ● Often associated with bile duct stones.

▶ **MRI findings**
A water-filled diverticulum appears as a hyperintense mass on the medial aspect of the duodenum on T2-weighted images ● After oral administration of an iron oxide contrast agent, the diverticulum loses its signal.

▶ **CT findings**
Outpouching of the duodenal lumen filled with air, fluid, or partially digested food ● The apparent size of the lesion can vary on follow-up investigations depending on the degree of filling.

▶ **Endoscopic findings**
Outpouching in the immediate vicinity of the papilla that can obscure the papilla ● A diverticulum with a very narrow neck may not be recognizable as such. ● After ERCP, the diverticulum often gets filled with contrast agent.

▶ **Upper gastrointestinal series**
Outpouching in the immediate vicinity of the papilla that fills with contrast agent.

Clinical Aspects

▶ **Typical presentation**
Usually asymptomatic ● The bile duct stones frequently associated with the disorder can themselves lead to symptoms ● Rarely, inflammation (diverticulitis) occurs with pain, fever, nausea, or vomiting.

▶ **Therapeutic options**
Surgery is indicated only to treat perforation or bleeding ● Ectopic bacterial colonization is managed with antibiotics.

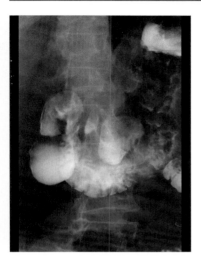

Fig. 6.3 Duodenal diverticulum. Upper gastrointestinal series. Large diverticulum in the ascending part of the duodenum.

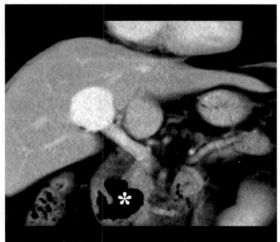

Fig. 6.4 Duodenal diverticulum. CT. Large juxtapapillary diverticulum (asterisk) that communicates with the duodenal lumen. Other findings include a large hypervascular mass in the hilum of the liver (aneurysm of the portal vein).

► **Course and prognosis**
Usually uncomplicated.
► **What does the clinician want to know?**
Exclude a tumor.

Differential Diagnosis

Pseudocyst of the pancreas	– Dilated or irregular pancreatic duct
	– Clinical picture of pancreatitis
Cystic pancreatic tumor	– Multicystic or septated
	– Pseudocyst remains unchanged after oral administration of an iron oxide contrast agent
Perforated duodenal ulcer	– Fluid and signs of inflammation around the ulcer
	– Pneumoperitoneum

Tips and Pitfalls

Lesion can be misinterpreted as a pancreatic pseudocyst or cystic tumor of the head of the pancreas.

Selected Literature

Cem Balci N et al. Juxtapapillary diverticulum. Findings on CT and MRI. Clin Imag 2003; 27: 82–88

Macari M et al. Duodenal diverticula mimicking cystic neoplasm of the pancreas: CT and MR imaging findings in seven patients. AJR 2003; 180: 195–199

Mazziotti S et al. MR cholangiopancreatography diagnosis of juxtapapillary duodenal diverticulum simulating a cystic lesion of the pancreas: usefulness of an oral negative contrast agent. AJR 2005; 185: 432–435

Definition

Saccular outpouching of the ileum resulting from a persistent vitelline duct.

▶ **Epidemiology**
Most common congenital anomaly of the gastrointestinal tract ● Prevalence is 1–3%.

▶ **Etiology, pathophysiology, pathogenesis**
Incomplete involution of the vitelline duct ● In 50% of cases, the lesion contains ectopic tissue (usually gastric mucosa) in addition to ileal mucosa.

Imaging Signs

▶ **Modality of choice**
Enteroclysis, CT.

▶ **Pathognomonic findings**
Ileal diverticulum with a length of 4–10 cm ● Located at a distance up to 100 cm from the ileocecal valve (usually 50–60 cm).
Complications: Bleeding from ectopic gastric mucosa ● Small bowel obstruction ● Diverticulitis ● Invagination ● Volvulus ● Herniation (Littré hernia).

▶ **Enteroclysis**
Saccular, blind outpouching of the ileum ● Usually in the right lower abdomen or pelvis ● Wide opening or with a narrow neck ● Occasionally exhibits filling defects due to foreign bodies or enteroliths.

▶ **CT findings**
Indicated in acute abdomen ● Even when a Meckel diverticulum causing obstruction or other complication is not detectable, the location and acute situation will be obvious ● Occasionally the diverticulum is detectable by these signs—fluid level or filled with fecal material ● An enterolith can often be demonstrated in diverticulitis ● Multidetector CT is also indicated in severe bleeding.

▶ **Ultrasound findings**
Important diagnostic modality, especially in children ● Round or long cystic structure ● Thick, hyperechoic inner wall ● Hypoechoic outer wall.

▶ **Angiographic findings**
Severe bleeding leads to extravasation of contrast agent ● Bleeding should prompt a search for a vitelline artery.

▶ **Findings on nuclear medicine imaging**
A lesion containing gastric mucosa is visualized as a small round area of increased focal uptake in the right lower abdomen (less sensitive in adults than in children).

▶ **Capsule endoscopy**
Recommended in adults with occult bleeding.

Fig. 7.1 Saccular Meckel diverticulum in a loop of the terminal ileum. Enteroclysis.

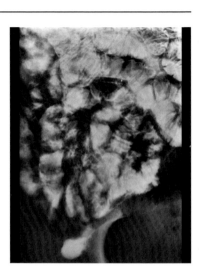

Clinical Aspects

▶ **Typical presentation**
Usually asymptomatic ● About a third of cases are diagnosed due to complications ● Often occurs within the first 10 years of life.
Complications: Bleeding from the middle of the gastrointestinal tract ● Painful small bowel obstruction ● Pain, fever, and vomiting occur in diverticulitis.

▶ **Therapeutic options**
Surgical resection.

▶ **Course and prognosis**
The risk of complications is 4% up to the age of 20 years, 2% up to the age of 40 years, and approaches zero in advanced age ● Tumors very rarely occur in diverticula in advanced age (usually carcinoids).

▶ **What does the clinician want to know?**
Is a Meckel diverticulum the cause of gastrointestinal bleeding?

Differential Diagnosis

Appendicitis	– Immediately adjacent to the cecum
	– Not compressible on ultrasound
Diverticulitis on the right side	– Pericolic inflammation
	– Colonic diverticulum
	– Thickened colonic wall
Acquired diverticulum	– Often multiple diverticula

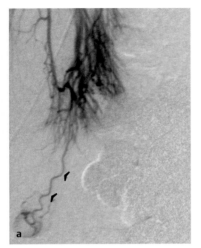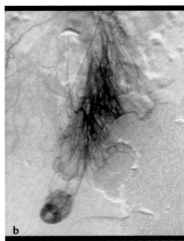

Fig. 7.2a,b Meckel diverticulum. DSA. Image demonstrates vitelline artery (arrowheads **a**). Late arterial phase (**b**). The diverticulum is well perfused.

Pseudodiverticula (sacculations in Crohn disease)	– Thickened small and large bowel loops – Proliferation of fatty and fibrotic tissue ("creeping fat") – Fistulas
Lymphoma or gastrointestinal stromal tumor	– Bowel wall is usually thickened – Continuous with the normal bowel lumen without outpouching

Tips and Pitfalls

Errors include failing to search for a vitelline artery (CT angiography may be helpful).

Selected Literature

Bennet GL et al. CT of Meckel's diverticulitis in 11 patients. AJR 2004; 182: 625–629

Levy AD et al. Meckel diverticulum: radiologic features with pathologic correlation. RadioGraphics 2004; 24: 565–587

Mitchell AW et al. Meckel's diverticulum: angiographic findings in 16 patients. AJR 1998; 170: 1329–1333

Definition

▶ **Epidemiology**
   Third most common small bowel tumor • Accounts for 10–15% of all small bowel tumors • Most often occurs between the ages of 40 and 60 years and in children.
▶ **Etiology, pathophysiology, pathogenesis**
   Most cases (95%) involve non-Hodgkin lymphoma of the B-cell phenotype • About 5% are peripheral T-cell lymphomas • Non-Hodgkin lymphomas primarily arise in the stomach (50%); small bowel (35%), colon (15%), and esophagus (< 1%) • Small bowel lesions occur primarily in the ileum • T-cell lymphomas occur more often in the duodenum and jejunum; they show less pronounced thickening of the wall and more often lead to perforations.

Imaging Signs

▶ **Modality of choice**
   CT, enteroclysis.
▶ **Pathognomonic findings**
   – *Infiltrative form:* Accounts for up to 50% of all lesions • Often there is a long segment of thickened bowel wall • Mucosal destruction • Obstruction is rare • Paradoxical dilation of the lumen in the affected segment.
   – *Polypoid form:* Isolated or multiple polyps distributed within the bowel wall • Ulcerations are occasionally present • Can lead to invagination • Rarely obstructive.
   – *Nodular form:* Multiple submucosal nodules.
   – *Exophytic form:* Extensive ulcerations • Leads to cavitations outside the bowel lumen.
   – *Mesenteric form:* Infiltration of adjacent bowel loops • Encasement of mesenteric vascular structures • Retroperitoneal lymph nodes are enlarged.
▶ **CT findings**
   – *Infiltrative form:* Thickened wall without layering • Only slight contrast enhancement • Lumen is often dilated.
   – *Polypoid form:* Nodular masses of varying size.
   – *Nodular form:* Only detectable once nodules are larger than 1–2 cm.
   – *Mesenteric form:* Usually there are several mesenteric nodules encasing vascular structures • Occasionally with streaky or patchy infiltration into the surrounding fatty tissue.
▶ **Findings on enteroclysis**
   – *Infiltrative form:* Thickened wall without the normal relief of the folds • Lumen is often dilated.
   – *Polypoid form:* Polypoid masses of varying size.
   – *Nodular form:* Nodular mucosal structure.
   – *Mesenteric form:* Displacement or compression of small bowel loops.
▶ **Ultrasound findings**
   Hypoechoic thickened bowel wall • Absence of peristalsis • Enlarged lymph nodes.

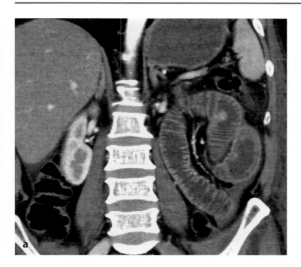

Fig. 7.3 a, b
Lymphoma of the small bowel. CT.
a Slight uniform thickening of the wall in an upper ileal loop.
b Long segment of thickened wall in a loop of the terminal ileum with ascitic fluid in the pelvis.

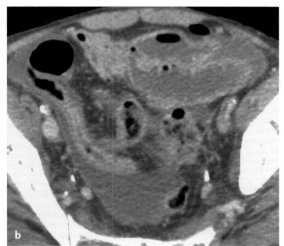

Fig. 7.4 Burkitt lymphoma of the small bowel. MR image. Long segment of thickened bowel wall in the ileum.

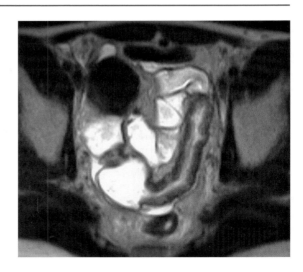

Clinical Aspects

▶ **Typical presentation**
This depends on the size and location of the primary tumor ● Diarrhea ● Weight loss ● Uncharacteristic pain ● Fever.

▶ **Therapeutic options**
Surgical removal ● Chemotherapy ● Radiation therapy.

▶ **Course and prognosis**
Prognosis is better than for small-bowel carcinoma.

▶ **What does the clinician want to know?**
Exclude an inflammatory bowel disorder such as Crohn disease.

Differential Diagnosis

Carcinoma of the small bowel	– Occurs more often in the jejunum – Circular growth pattern with obstructive symptoms – Not as well perfused
Crohn disease	– Leads to strictures – Fistulas – Acutely inflamed wall shows marked contrast enhancement
Gastrointestinal stromal tumor	– Often large exophytic tumors – With central necrotic areas

Tips and Pitfalls
....

Can be misdiagnosed as Crohn disease.

Selected Literature

Buckley JA et al. Small bowel cancer: imaging features and staging. Radiol Clin North Am 1997; 35: 381–402

Byun JH et al. CT findings in peripheral T-cell lymphoma involving the gastrointestinal tract. Radiology 2003; 227: 59–67

Horton KM et al. Multidetector-row computed tomography and 3-dimensional computed tomography imaging of small bowel neoplasms. Current concept in diagnosis. J Comput Assist Tomogr 2004; 28: 106–116

Definition

▶ **Epidemiology**
This is the cause of 10–20% of acute abdomen cases ● Small bowel obstruction is much more common than colonic obstruction, accounting for 75% of all cases.

▶ **Etiology, pathophysiology, pathogenesis**
Adhesion (50–80%) ● Hernia (10–15%) ● Tumor (10–15%) ● Crohn disease ● Intussusception ● Volvulus ● Endometriosis ● Gall stones ● Hematoma.

Imaging Signs

▶ **Modality of choice**
Plain abdominal radiography ● Multidetector CT (in acute abdomen).

▶ **Pathognomonic findings**
Dilated small bowel loops (> 2.5 cm) ● Filled with fluid and gas ● Abrupt transitions between dilated and collapsed bowel loops ● Differences in perfusion in strangulation ● Obstruction of venous drainage (most common cause of ischemia) ● Fluid or streaky changes in the mesentery ● Pneumoperitoneum in perforation.

▶ **Findings on plain abdominal radiography**
Dilated small bowel loops with fluid levels ● Little air and fecal material in the colon ● Normal findings in one-third of the bowel ● Isolated obstruction is indistinguishable from strangulation with bowel ischemia.

▶ **CT findings**
Modality of choice in a high-grade obstruction or serious clinical picture ● Demonstrates the cause in 90–95% of cases ● Ischemia can be diagnosed with relative certainty (sensitivity is 90%) ● Transitional zones and rare causes of obstruction are well visualized ● Direct visualization of an adhesion is unusual (diagnosis is made by exclusion) ● Oral contrast administration is not required in high-grade obstruction as air and fluid provide sufficient contrast ● Intravenous contrast administration is required to evaluate perfusion of the bowel loops.

▶ **MRI**
Alternative to CT in very young patients and pregnant women.

▶ **Ultrasound findings**
Indicated in children and adolescents ● Usually inconclusive in adults with intensely painful acute abdomen.

▶ **Upper gastrointestinal series and enteroclysis**
Not indicated in high-grade obstruction.

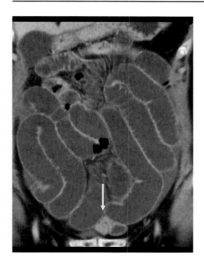

Fig. 7.5 Ileus from adhesions. CT. Dilated and fluid-filled small bowel loops. Obstruction and transition from abnormal to normal bowel in the center of the lower abdomen (arrow).

Clinical Aspects

▶ **Typical presentation**
Crampy upper abdominal pain ● Muscular rigidity in the abdomen ● The preoperative diagnosis of strangulation is unreliable in over 50% of cases.

▶ **Therapeutic options**
Immediate surgical intervention is indicated in high-grade obstruction and ischemia ● A gastric tube is indicated in less severe cases.

▶ **Course and prognosis**
Mortality is about 1–2% ● Complications include ischemia and perforation, which markedly increase morbidity and mortality.

▶ **What does the clinician want to know?**
Is there an obstruction? ● If yes, determine the cause, level, and extent of the obstruction.

Differential Diagnosis

Paralytic ileus	– Dilated small and large bowel loops
	– No transitional zone
	– No other cause of obstruction

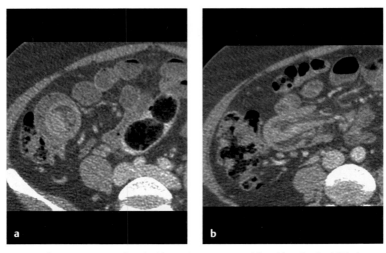

Fig. 7.6 a, b   Invagination of an ileal loop. CT. Transverse (**a**) and longitudinal (**b**) views.

Tips and Pitfalls

Errors include late realization that CT is indicated ● The result is an arduous diagnosis process involving upper gastrointestinal series or enteroclysis.

Selected Literature

Aufort S et al. Multidetector CT of bowel obstruction: value of post-processing. Eur Radiol 1997; 15: 625–636

Maglinte DDT et al. Current concepts of small bowel obstruction. Radiol Clin North Am 2003; 41: 263–283

Taourel P et al. Non-traumatic abdominal emergencies: imaging of acute intestinal obstruction. Eur Radiol 2002; 12: 2151–2160

Definition

Pericolic inflammation secondary to microscopic or macroscopic perforation of a colonic diverticulum (peridiverticulitis). Modified Hinchey classification:

- *Stage Ia:* Circumscribed pericolic inflammation.
- *Stage Ib:* Circumscribed pericolic abscess (< 3 cm).
- *Stage II:* Larger abscess in the pelvis or retroperitoneum.
- *Stage III:* Suppurative peritonitis.
- *Stage IV:* Macroscopic perforation with fecal peritonitis.

► **Epidemiology**

Diverticulosis (presence of diverticula) occurs in 5–10% of people over 45 years and in 50–60% of people over 80 years. Up to 20% of patients with diverticulitis are younger than 50 years. Symptoms occur in 20% of cases. There is no sex predilection. 85% of all inflammations occur in the sigmoid and descending colon.

► **Etiology, pathophysiology, pathogenesis**

Increased intraluminal pressure and weakness of the bowel wall ● This leads to herniation of the mucosa and muscularis mucosa (pseudodiverticulum) at the weak point where the vasa recta enter the colon ● Fecal matter is retained in the diverticula ● Mucosal inflammation ● Diverticulitis invariably arises from a microscopic perforation.

Imaging Signs

► **Modality of choice**

CT ● Ultrasound (in mild cases).

► **Pathognomonic findings**

Diverticula (indicators of disease) ● Inflammatory changes in the pericolic fatty tissue ● Thickening of the wall of the colon (usually over a long segment) ● Intramural or pericolic abscesses (prognostic sign) ● Fistulas (usually to the bladder) ● Bowel obstruction ● Free air (rare).

► **CT findings**

Bowel wall is thickened ● Densities in the surrounding fatty tissue ● Thickened fascia ● Abscesses ● Pericolic fluid collections ● Free air at the site of macroscopic perforation.

► **Ultrasound findings**

Thickened, hypoechoic segment of the colon ● Diverticula (hypoechoic or hyperechoic paracolic focal lesions) ● Poorly demarcated hypoechoic areas around the inflamed diverticula ● Inflamed region is tender to palpation.

► **MRI findings**

Hypointense thickened wall on T1-weighted images ● The spread of the pericolic inflammation can be readily evaluated on T2-weighted images with fat suppression by observing the hyperintense edema ● The inflamed, thickened wall enhances with contrast (indicated in younger patients and pregnant women).

► **Contrast enema**

Increasingly replaced by other modalities as it only permits a rough estimate of the extent of the pericolic inflammation.

Fig. 8.1 a, b Diverticulitis of the sigmoid.
a Contrast enema. Long segment of a
high-grade stenosis of the sigmoid colon.
b CT. Severe thickening of the bowel wall
with a small anterior abscess within the
bowel wall.

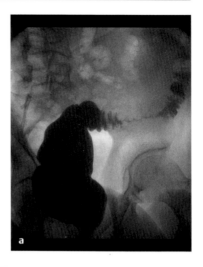

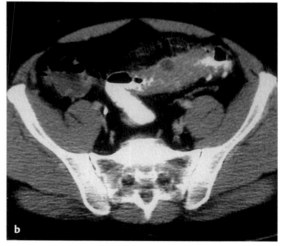

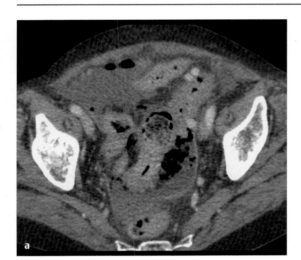

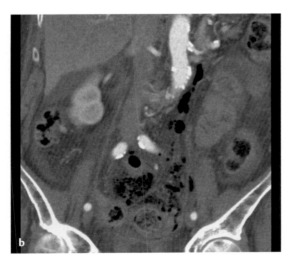

Fig. 8.2 a, b Acute diverticulitis with macroscopic perforation. Pericolic collection of fluid and gas (**a**). The gas can be traced back into the retroperitoneal space to the origin of the left renal artery (**b**).

▶ **Endoscopy**
Painful in the acute stage • Not very helpful from a diagnostic standpoint as it does not allow evaluation of the extraluminal inflammation.

Clinical Aspects
....

▶ **Typical presentation**
Pain in the left lower abdomen • Fever • Leukocytosis • Tenderness to palpation • Occasionally there is a palpable tumor • Pneumaturia, feces in the urine, and/or recurrent urinary tract infections are indicators of a colovesical fistula • Bleeding is a complication of diverticulosis but not diverticulitis.

▶ **Therapeutic options**
Antibiotic treatment is sufficient for mild forms • Severe forms (20% of cases) require surgery • Certain cases may require percutaneous abscess drainage • Surgery is indicated in generalized peritonitis or sepsis and in immunocompromised patients.

▶ **Course and prognosis**
Seventy percent of cases are mild forms that respond well to conservative treatment • Severe forms have a mortality of 2–5% • More severe clinical courses occur in younger patients • In renal insufficiency and immunosuppression, symptoms are less pronounced, macroscopic perforations are common, and postoperative morbidity and mortality are increased.

▶ **What does the clinician want to know?**
How severe is the inflammation? This determines whether conservative, surgical, or interventional treatment is indicated.

Differential Diagnosis

Carcinoma of the colon	– History: Insidious onset, often with blood in the stool – No signs of inflammation – Short segment of thickened bowel wall (often more than 2 cm), often eccentric – Fewer pericolic changes and no fascial thickening
Inflammatory bowel disease	– No pericolic changes in ulcerative colitis – Usually small bowel involvement or discontinuous involvement in Crohn disease
Ischemic colitis	– Long segment of uniformly thickened bowel wall, usually in the area supplied by the inferior mesenteric artery – Slight pericolic reaction – Pneumatosis in advanced cases
Appendicitis	– Pain on the lower right side – Appendicitis demonstrated by ultrasound
Inflammation of the epiploic appendices	– Pericolic round fatty nodules with an inflammatory halo

Tips and Pitfalls

Can be misinterpreted as a tumor.

Selected Literature

Ambrosetti P et al. Colonic diverticulitis: impact of imaging on surgical management—a prospective study of 542 patients. Eur Radiol 2002; 12: 1145–1149

Kaiser AM et al. The management of complicated diverticulitis and the role of computed tomography. Am J Gastroenterol 2005; 100: 910–917

Kircher MF et al. Frequency, sensitivity, and specificity of individual signs of diverticulitis on thin-section helical CT with colonic contrast material: experience with 312 cases. AJR 2002; 178: 1313–1318

Colon and Anus

Definition

Chronic inflammatory disorder of the colon limited to the mucosa.

▶ **Epidemiology**

Usually manifests itself between the ages of 20 and 40 years; second age peak is in elderly patients ● Slightly more common in women ● Prevalence shows great regional variation: it is higher in Europe, the United States, and Australia than in other parts of the world.

▶ **Etiology, pathophysiology, pathogenesis**

Etiology is unclear; postulated causes include infection, allergy to food components, and immune reaction to bacteria or bacterial antigens ● There is a genetic predisposition ● The lesion begins immediately behind the anal ring ● Spreads continuously and cranially ● Proctosigmoiditis occurs in 40–50% of cases, left-sided colitis in 30%, subtotal colitis (up to the right colic flexure), and pancolitis in 20% ● A compromised ileocecal valve can promote spread of inflammation to the terminal ileum as backwash ileitis.

Imaging Signs

▶ **Modality of choice**

Endoscopy, ultrasound, MR enteroclysis.

▶ **Pathognomonic findings**

Bowel wall is thickened to over 3 mm in the distended state ● Bowel shows marked enhancement in the active phase ● Absence of haustration creates a tubelike appearance.

Complications: Toxic megacolon (diameter exceeding 5–6 cm) ● Perforation ● Scarred stricture ● Carcinoma of the colon ● Associated with primary sclerosing cholangitis in 3% of cases.

▶ **Endoscopic findings**

Satinlike, finely granular mucosal surface ● Friable surface that bleeds when touched with the endoscope ● Mucosal ulcerations ● After healing, the colon appears tubelike with atrophic mucosa and inflammatory pseudopolyps.

▶ **Ultrasound findings**

Important as the primary diagnostic modality ● Thickening of the bowel wall, which in the florid stage is highly perfused (demonstrated by color Doppler and ultrasound contrast agents) ● Peristalsis is reduced in the thickened bowel segments ● Stenoses are clearly visualized.

▶ **Findings on plain abdominal radiography**

Useful in demonstrating toxic megacolon (diameter exceeding 5–6 cm) ● Bowel wall may show irregular thickening ● No feces in the colon.

▶ **Findings on contrast enema**

Fine mucosal granular pattern ● Ulcerations are usually limited to the mucosal surface but occasionally undermine the mucosa and extend as far as the muscularis ("collar button ulcers") ● Later, round or long pseudopolyps create filling defects ● This modality has largely been superseded by endoscopy.

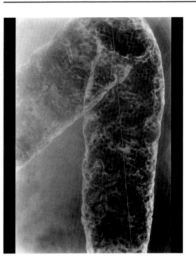

Fig. 8.3 Late phase of ulcerative colitis. Double contrast. Loss of haustration and multiple round to oblong pseudopolyps at the splenic flexure of the colon.

► **CT findings**
Thickening of the bowel wall • Marked enhancement after contrast administration in the florid stage of inflammation • The stenoses (usually covering long segments) are well visualized. *Indications:* primarily in the presence of complications, especially perforation.

► **MRI findings**
Only a supplementary modality • Bowel wall is thickened • On fat-suppressed T2-weighted images, the acute inflammation (edema) is well visualized, with an intense signal in the bowel wall and vicinity • Good modality for visualizing stenoses.

Clinical Aspects

► **Typical presentation**
Perianal bleeding • Bloody diarrhea • Cramps • Frequent abdominal pain. *Extraintestinal symptoms:* Arthropathy of the major joints (5–10%) • Episcleritis and uveitis • Erythema nodosum • Pyoderma gangrenosum (1–2%) • Primary sclerosing cholangitis (3%) • Ankylosing spondylitis.

► **Therapeutic options**
Primary topical treatment with 5-aminosalicylic acid or corticoid enemas • Corticoids or immunosuppressive agents are indicated in severe cases • Surgery is required in 20–30% of all patients to manage treatment-resistant disease, perforation, or toxic megacolon.

Fig. 8.4 a, b
Ulcerative colitis.
MR image.
a Slight thickening
of the wall of the
ascending and
transverse colon
and local pseudo-
polypoid thickening
of the wall.
b The bowel wall
and pseudopoly-
poid lesions en-
hance with contrast.

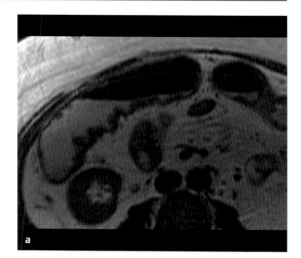

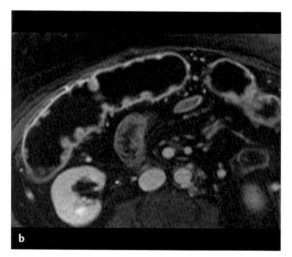

▶ **Course and prognosis**
Clinical course is highly variable ● High rate of recurrence (80%) ● Periods of remission can last from weeks to years ● 10–15% of patients experience a chronic active clinical course ● Only 1% experience just a single episode ● Risk of carcinoma of the colon increases with long periods of high disease activity.

▶ **What does the clinician want to know?**
Exclude other inflammatory or ischemic disorders of the bowel ● Extent ● Severity ● Complications.

Differential Diagnosis

Crohn disease	– Usually associated with small bowel involvement – Transmural inflammation with fistulas and abscesses – Proliferation of fatty and fibrotic tissue ("creeping fat") – Spreads from the terminal ileum toward the rectum
Ischemic colitis	– Older patients – Vascular pathology – Reduced perfusion of the bowel wall
Diverticulitis	– Diverticula – Circumscribed thickening of the bowel wall – Pericolic inflammation in fatty tissue – Thickening of the fascia – Usually limited to the sigmoid colon
Pseudomembranous colitis	– Complication of antibiotics and cytostatic agents – Bowel wall thickening is usually more pronounced than in bowel disorders – Marked enhancement of the mucosa after contrast administration

Tips and Pitfalls

Collapsed bowel loops can mimic thickening of the bowel wall.

Selected Literature

Carucci LR et al. Radiographic imaging in inflammatory bowel disease. Gastroenterol Clin North Am 2002; 31: 93–117

Gore RM et al. CT features in ulcerative colitis and Crohn's disease. AJR 1996; 167: 3–15

Horton KM et al. CT evaluation of the colon: inflammatory disease. RadioGraphics 2000; 20: 399–418

Definition

Inflammatory disorder of the colon that occurs as a complication of antibiotic treatment.

▶ **Epidemiology**

Humans represent the main reservoir of *Clostridium difficile*, which is not part of the normal intestinal flora • The pathogen occurs in 2–3% of healthy adults and in 5–15% of asymptomatic inpatients and outpatients.

▶ **Etiology, pathophysiology, pathogenesis**

Infection with *C. difficile* is a hospital-acquired infection that usually occurs secondary to antibiotic treatment • Further predisposing factors include immunosuppression, chemotherapy, intensive care, and major surgery • The disorder is caused by toxin produced by the pathogen • This leads to formation of pseudo-membranous, exudative, inflammatory plaques in the colon • Occasionally the small bowel is also involved.

Imaging Signs

▶ **Modality of choice**

Endoscopy, ultrasound, CT.

▶ **Pathognomonic findings**

Bowel wall is thickened owing to edema • Mucosa enhances markedly • The rest of the wall is thickened but does not enhance (edema) • Haustration is preserved • Usually there is only slight pericolic inflammation • The rectum and sigmoid colon are involved in 80–90% of cases • Segmental involvement is more common than diffuse involvement.

Complications: Toxic megacolon (diameter > 5–6 cm) • Perforation.

▶ **Endoscopic findings**

Cream-colored confluent plaques or pseudomembranes on fragile mucosa • Primarily located in the rectum and sigmoid colon • Lesions are occasionally limited to the ascending colon.

▶ **Ultrasound findings**

Thickening of the bowel wall, which in the florid stage is highly perfused (demonstrated by color Doppler and ultrasound contrast agents) • Peristalsis is reduced in the thickened bowel segments.

▶ **CT findings**

Swollen bowel wall • Occasionally several layers can be differentiated (target sign) • Mucosa enhances markedly with contrast • The edematous bowel wall does not enhance • Ascites may occur in very severe cases • Oral or rectal contrast agent is trapped between the swollen mucosal folds (accordion sign).

▶ **Findings on plain abdominal radiography**

Demonstrates toxic megacolon (diameter exceeding 5–6 cm) • Bowel wall occasionally appears irregularly thickened • No feces in the colon • The extent and severity of the disorder are often underestimated.

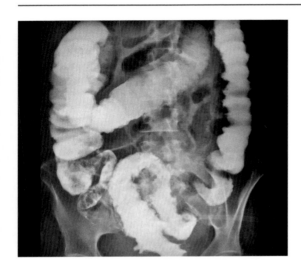

Fig. 8.5 Pseudo-membranous colitis. Single-contrast image of the colon. Irregular contour of the rectum and sigmoid.

▶ **Findings on contrast enema**
Largely replaced by endoscopy and cross-sectional imaging modalities • Pseudomembranous plaques cause small nodular filling defects • Confluent pseudomembranes produce a grossly irregular mucosal surface.

▶ **MRI findings**
Bowel wall is thickened • On fat-suppressed T2-weighted images, the acute inflammation (edema) is well visualized • There is an intense signal in the bowel wall and vicinity • Good modality for visualizing stenoses • However, MRI is only a supplementary modality.

Clinical Aspects

▶ **Typical presentation**
Broad spectrum of symptoms • Slight diarrhea may be present and cease after antibiotic treatment is discontinued • Any degree of severity is possible, including severe colitis with intense watery diarrhea (bloody in 10% of cases), abdominal cramps, and fever • Life-threatening complications can result from shock, bowel perforation, and megacolon • Acute abdomen or abdominal sepsis occurs in 5% of cases • Symptoms can begin immediately after the onset of antibiotic treatment or may only occur weeks later • Toxin is detected in the feces.

▶ **Therapeutic options**
Discontinue the antibiotics • Fluid and electrolyte substitution • Metronidazole and vancomycin may be indicated in severe cases.

Fig. 8.6 a–c
Pseudomembra-
nous colitis.
a CT. The entire
visualized segment
of the colon up to
the splenic flexure
exhibits marked
thickening of the
wall. The mucosa is
well perfused and
there is free fluid in
the lower abdomen.
b Ultrasound.
Thickened, hypo-
echoic wall at the
junction of the de-
scending colon and
sigmoid.

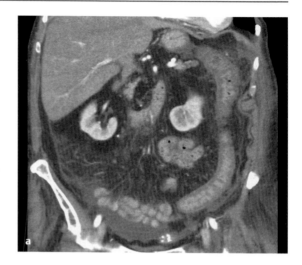

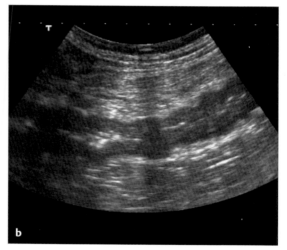

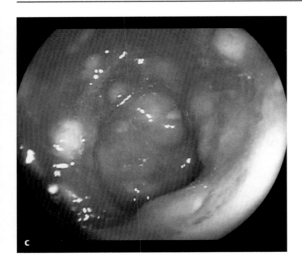

c Endoscopy. Typical yellow plaques on the surface of the mucosa.

▶ **Course and prognosis**
  Mortality is 1–3.5% ● Left untreated, the severe form has a mortality of 15–30%.
▶ **What does the clinician want to know?**
  Exclude ischemic disorders of the bowel ● Extent ● Severity ● Complications.

Differential Diagnosis

Ischemic colitis	– Older patients – Vascular pathology is present – Reduced perfusion of the bowel wall
Diverticulitis	– Diverticula – Pericolic inflammation in fatty tissue – Thickening of the fascia – Usually most pronounced in the sigmoid colon
Crohn disease	– Usually associated with small bowel involvement – Transmural inflammation with fistulas and abscesses – Proliferation of fatty and fibrotic tissue ("creeping fat) – Spreads from the terminal ileum toward the rectum
Simple antibiotic-associated colitis	– Watery (not bloody) diarrhea that ceases spontaneously when drug is discontinued – No plaques or membranes

Tips and Pitfalls
....

Normal CT findings do not exclude *Clostridium* colitis ● Conversely, severe morphologic changes correlate poorly with the clinical picture.

Selected Literature

Ash L et al. Colonic abnormalities on CT in adult hospitalised patients with clostridium difficile colitis: prevalence and significance of findings. AJR 2006; 186: 1393–1400

Kawamoto S et al. Pseudomembraneous colitis: spectrum of imaging findings with clinical and pathological correlation. RadioGraphics 1999; 19: 887–897

Kirkpatrick IDC, Greenberg HM: Evaluating the CT diagnosis of clostridium difficile colitis: should CT guide therapy? AJR 2001; 176: 635–639

Definition

Acute inflammation of the appendix due to obstruction of the lumen.

▶ **Epidemiology**

The lifetime risk of developing acute appendicitis is about 7% • Occurs in all age groups • Slightly more common in males • Most common indication for surgery in children.

▶ **Etiology, pathophysiology, pathogenesis**

Obstruction of the lumen of the appendix • This leads to distension, inflammation, and finally perforation.

Imaging Signs

▶ **Modality of choice**

Ultrasound • CT where a perforation is suspected.

▶ **Pathognomonic findings**

Distended appendix with bull's eye appearance (diameter > 7 mm) • Blind fingerlike end • Thickened wall (> 3 mm) • Appendicolith • Pericecal fluid or infiltration of fatty tissue

▶ **Ultrasound findings**

Distended appendix appears as a hypoechoic double-layered band • Careful compression produces pain over the appendix • A hypoechoic, inhomogeneously structured area in the region of the appendix suggests perforation with a perityphlic abscess • Increased signal on color Doppler studies • Air in the appendix is inconsistent with acute inflammation • Retrocecal appendicitis can be masked by overlying air • Accuracy for an experienced examiner is over 90%, and the rate of appendectomy with negative findings can be considerably reduced compared with clinical examination alone.

▶ **CT findings**

Thickened appendix with inflammatory infiltration of the surrounding fatty tissue • An appendicolith is visualized in 30–40% of cases • Ileus is present in the terminal ileum in severe inflammation or perforation • After intravenous administration of contrast, the inflamed appendix is better demarcated • CT is superior to ultrasound for imaging perforations, especially of a retrocecal appendix.

▶ **MRI findings**

Thickened appendix • Appendix and inflamed surrounding tissue enhance markedly after intravenous contrast administration, especially with fat suppression • A perforation with abscess is demonstrated particularly well • Indicated in pregnant women and young patients where ultrasound is insufficient.

Fig. 8.7 a, b Appendicitis. Ultrasound. Thickened wall and enlarged diameter of the appendix on longitudinal (**a**) and transverse (**b**) sections.

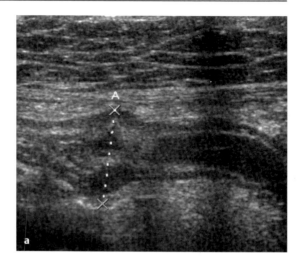

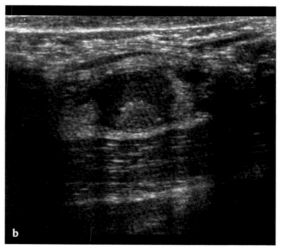

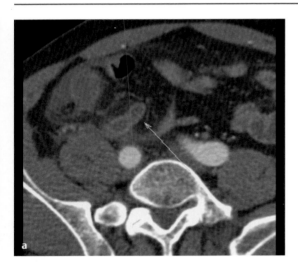

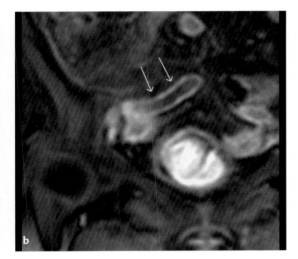

Fig. 8.8 a, b
Appendicitis. Enlarged, markedly enhancing appendix on CT (**a**) and MR image (**b**).

Fig. 8.9 a, b Perforated appendix with abscess in appendicitis. MR image.
a Abscess on the roof of the bladder (asterisk).
b Thickened, enhancing appendix communicating with the abscess (arrow).

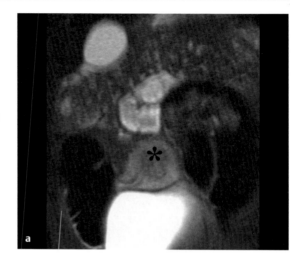

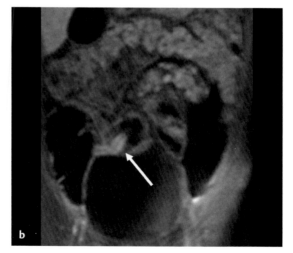

Clinical Aspects

▶ **Typical presentation**
Periumbilical pain that migrates into the right lower abdomen ● Nausea ● Vomiting ● Fever ● McBurney point is tender to palpation ● Imaging studies are important as only 60% of patients present with the classic clinical picture.

▶ **Therapeutic options**
Appendectomy • Larger abscesses may require percutaneous drainage in certain cases.
▶ **Course and prognosis**
Prognosis is good with timely surgical intervention without postoperative complications.
▶ **What does the clinician want to know?**
Is this appendicitis (an indication for surgery), or is the acute abdominal pain attributable to another cause that may be treated conservatively?

Differential Diagnosis

Mesenteric lymphadenitis	– Enlarged lymph nodes
	– Slight thickening of the wall of the terminal ileum and cecum
Crohn disease	– Longer medical history
	– Significant thickening of the wall of the terminal ileum
	– Reduced peristalsis in the terminal ileum
	– Thickened bowel wall enhances
Oophoritis	– Normal-sized appendix
	– Area over the gonads is tender to palpation with an applicator
Tumor of the appendix	– Chronic symptoms
	– Irregular thickening of the bowel wall spreading to the cecum
Cecal diverticulitis	– Diverticula in the ascending colon
	– Peridiverticulitis in the fatty tissue
	– Circumscribed thickening of the wall of the cecum
Inflammation of the epiploic appendices	– Pericolic round fatty nodules with an inflammatory halo

Tips and Pitfalls

A diameter over 7 mm should not be regarded as the sole sign of appendicitis • The collapsed ileum can be misinterpreted as the appendix.

Selected Literature

Keyzer C et al. Comparison of US and unenhanced multi-detector row CT in patients suspected of having acute appendicitis. Radiology 2005; 236: 527–534

Pinto Leite N et al. CT evaluation of appendicitis and its complications: imaging techniques and key diagnostic findings AJR 2005; 185: 406–417

Rao PM et al. Helical CT for the diagnosis of appendicitis: prospective evaluation of a focused appendix CT examination. Radiology 2002; 202: 139–144

Definition

Projections of mucosa into the bowel lumen that can degenerate into malignancies.

▶ **Epidemiology**
Approximately 10% of the population have polyps • Prevalence increases with age.

▶ **Etiology, pathophysiology, pathogenesis**
Smaller polyps are often hyperplastic polyps • Larger polyps (> 1 cm) are more likely to be adenomas • Approximately 90% of colorectal carcinomas develop from adenomas (adenoma-carcinoma sequence) • The risk of carcinoma increases with size (1 cm: < 1%; 1–2 cm: 5–10%; over 2 cm: about 10–50%) • Other criteria for increased risk of cancer include three or more adenomas, the degree of dysplasia, and the extent of villous tissue in the polyp • Flat adenomas of the depressed type are a special form; they become malignant early and metastasize.

Imaging Signs

▶ **Modality of choice**
Endoscopy, CT colonography.

▶ **Pathognomonic findings**
Polypoid mucosal changes • Pediculate or broad-based • Bowel wall is of normal thickness.

▶ **Endoscopic findings**
Macroscopic findings can often be correlated with histologic forms • Forceps biopsy and snare-loop polypectomy are possible • CT colonography is indicated when endoscopy is incomplete.

▶ **CT colonographic findings**
Polypoid lesions in the bowel wall • CT detects lesions measuring 3 mm or larger • Adenomas can enhance.

▶ **MR colonography**
Polypoid lesions in the bowel wall • MR detects lesions measuring 5 mm or larger • These lesions usually enhance markedly whereas hyperplastic polyps do not.

▶ **Double contrast studies**
No longer used as an imaging modality for diagnosing polyps.

Clinical Aspects

▶ **Typical presentation**
Usually asymptomatic • Blood in the stool is an early sign.

▶ **Therapeutic options**
Snare-loop polypectomy • Large flat polyps occasionally require surgical removal.

▶ **Course and prognosis**
Complete resection effectively prevents carcinoma • There is a high probability of recurrence in risk groups.

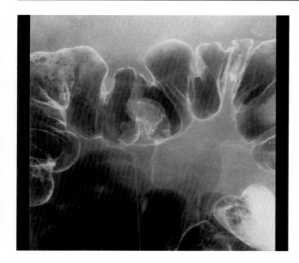

Fig. 8.10 Adenomatous polyp of the colon. Double-contrast study of the colon. Polypoid filling defect in the sigmoid colon.

► **What does the clinician want to know?**

Are clinically relevant polyps present (in gastroenterologic literature 1 cm or larger, in radiologic literature 6–8 mm or larger)?

Differential Diagnosis

Hyperplastic polyp	– Usually smaller than 1 cm
	– Does not enhance on MR image
Inflammatory pseudopolyp	– Associated with chronic inflammatory bowel disease
Mesenchymal polyp	– Often large
	– Intramural
	– Extraintestinal component
Diverticula	– Extraintestinal location is usually apparent
	– Hyperdense ring on unenhanced CT
Residual fecal matter	– Contains air
	– Changes position
	– Does not enhance with contrast

Tips and Pitfalls

Errors include poor preparation and insufficient insufflation of the bowel with air or CO_2.

Selected Literature

Hartmann D et al. Colorectal polyps: detection with dark-lumen MR colonography versus conventional colonoscopy. Radiology 2006; 238: 143–149

Fig. 8.11 a, b
Polyp fills the lumen.
MR image.
a VIBE sequence.
b Polyp enhances
markedly with con-
trast.

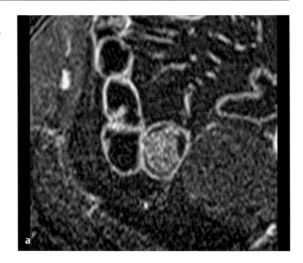

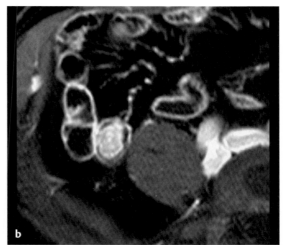

Macari M et al. Filling defects at CT colonography: Pseudo- and diminutive lesions (the good), polyps (the bad), flat lesions, masses, and carcinomas (the ugly). RadioGraphics 2003; 23: 1073–1091

Mulhall BP et al. Meta-analysis. Computed tomographic colonography. Ann Intern Med 2005; 142: 635–650

Definition

Malignant tumor of the mucosa of the colon • *Distribution:* Rectum (30%), sigmoid colon (45%), descending colon (10%), transverse and ascending colon (15%) • Metastasizes to regional lymph nodes and the liver.

▶ **Epidemiology**

Incidence increases with age • Most tumors occur after 50 years of age • Lifetime risk of disease is 6% • Second most common tumor in men and women • Risk factors include a low-fiber, high-protein, and high-fat diet and obesity.

▶ **Etiology, pathophysiology, pathogenesis**

About 90% of carcinomas arise from adenomatous polyps • A carcinoma is thought to take 10 years to develop.

Risk groups: Risk is doubled in immediate relatives of tumor patients • Persons genetically predisposed to hereditary colorectal carcinoma (familial adenomatous polyposis, hereditary nonpolypoid carcinoma of the colon) • Patients with chronic inflammatory bowel disease.

Imaging Signs

▶ **Modality of choice**

Endoscopy, CT.

▶ **Pathognomonic findings**

Irregular mucosal surface • Concentric thickening of the bowel wall • Lumen is narrowed • Large tumors show infiltration of the surrounding fatty tissue • Lymph node metastases.

▶ **Endoscopic findings**

Irregular mucosa with necrotic exophytic tumor • Modality permits biopsy • Gold standard for initial examination.

▶ **CT findings**

Circumscribed thickening of the bowel wall with narrowing of the lumen • The thickened bowel wall enhances with contrast • Lymph node involvement usually presents as involvement of multiple nodes rather than enlargement • CT colonography provides most information with intravenous contrast, for example immediately after colonoscopy discontinued due to tumor stenosis.

▶ **MRI findings**

Circumscribed thickening of the bowel wall with narrowing of the lumen • The thickened bowel wall occasionally enhances markedly with contrast • Affected lymph nodes, although often not noticeably enlarged, also show marked enhancement on fat-suppressed sequences.

▶ **Findings on contrast enema**

Now hardly ever used • Irregular contour of the mucosa • Lumen is narrowed.

▶ **PET or PET/CT findings**

Used in diagnosing recurrent tumors • Most reliable modality for demonstrating extraintestinal recurrent tumors in scar tissue.

Fig. 8.12 Carcinoma of the colon causing eccentric narrowing at the colic flexure. Double-contrast study.

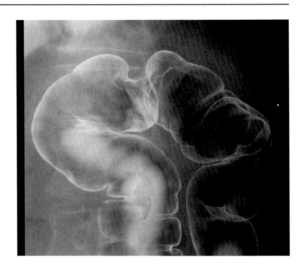

Clinical Aspects

▶ **Typical presentation**
  Remains asymptomatic for a long time • Changes in bowel habits • Anemia, pain, and weight loss are late symptoms.
▶ **Therapeutic options**
  Surgery.
▶ **Course and prognosis**
  Prognosis depends on the tumor stage • 5-year survival:
  – Dukes A (T1 N0 M0): 97–100%
  – Dukes B1 (T2 N0 M0): 82–90%
  – Dukes B2 (T3 N0 M0): 73–80%
  – Dukes B3 (T4 N0 M0): 63–75%
  – Dukes C (T1–4 N1–3 M0): 26–74%
▶ **What does the clinician want to know?**
  Location of the tumor • Tumor stage • Metastases.

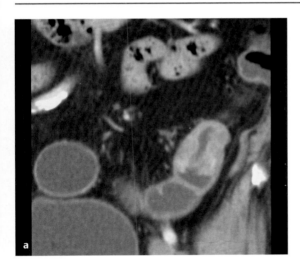

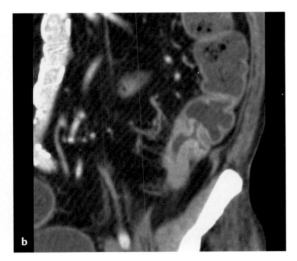

Fig. 8.13 a, b Carcinoma of the colon. CT. Circular thickening of the bowel wall with increased enhancement after contrast administration at the junction of the descending colon and sigmoid.

Differential Diagnosis

Diverticulitis	– Long segment of thickening of the bowel wall – Proved diverticula – Pericolic inflammation in adjacent fatty tissue – Thickening of the fascia
Ischemic colitis	– Long segment of thickened bowel wall – Reduced perfusion of the bowel wall – Occlusion or stenosis of arterial feeders
Ulcerative colitis	– Diffuse spread beginning in the rectum – Absence of haustration
Submucosal tumors (gastrointestinal stromal tumor, hemangioma)	– Eccentric narrowing of the lumen
Endometriosis	– External compression – Unilateral saw-tooth contour

Tips and Pitfalls

Insufficient filling of the colon with water or air on cross-sectional modalities is a common error.

Selected Literature

Cohade C et al. Direct comparison of (18)F-FDG PET and PET/CT in patients with colorectal carcinoma. J Nucl Me 2003; 44: 1797–1803

Fenlon HM et al. Occlusive colon carcinoma: virtual colonoscopy in the preoperative evaluation of the proximal colon. Radiology 1999; 210: 423–428

Horton KM et al. Spiral CT of colon cancer: cross sectional imaging and role in management. RadioGraphics 2000; 20: 419–430

Definition

Malignant tumor of the rectal mucosa.

▶ **Epidemiology**

Incidence increases with age • Lifetime risk of colorectal carcinoma is 6% • Usually occurs after 50 years.

▶ **Etiology, pathophysiology, pathogenesis**

About 90% of carcinomas arise from adenomatous polyps • *Risk groups:* Risk is doubled in immediate relatives of tumor patients; other risk groups include persons genetically predisposed to hereditary colorectal carcinoma (familial adenomatous polyposis, hereditary nonpolypoid carcinoma of the colon), and patients with chronic inflammatory bowel disease • Metastases occur in the regional lymph nodes (primary metastatic spread), lungs, and liver (secondary metastatic spread).

Imaging Signs

▶ **Modality of choice**

Endoscopy, MRI, endoscopic ultrasound.

▶ **Pathognomonic findings**

Irregular mucosal surface • Concentric thickening of the bowel wall • Lumen is narrowed • Large tumors show infiltration of the fatty tissue and mesorectum • Metastatic lymph nodes are often not enlarged.

▶ **Endoscopic findings**

Gold standard for initial examination • Irregular mucosa with necrotic exophytic tumor • Modality permits biopsy.

▶ **MRI findings**

T1-weighted images show a hypointense thickened bowel wall and a narrowed lumen • The extent of the tumor is well visualized on T2-weighted FSE sequences • Administration of intravenous contrast does not improve local staging compared with fat-suppressed sequences • Lymph node metastases are often small but multiple • Usually relationship of the tumor to the mesorectum is well visualized, more clearly than on endosonography.

▶ **Endoscopic ultrasound findings**

Very precisely visualizes the layers of the bowel • This makes it the method with the highest precision for the T classification, although quality decreases with increasing tumor size.

▶ **CT findings**

Significantly inferior to endoscopic ultrasound in T classification • Circumscribed thickening of the bowel wall with narrowing of the lumen • The thickened bowel wall enhances with contrast • Lymph node involvement more often presents as involvement of multiple nodes rather than enlargement.

Fig. 8.14 a, b
Malignant polypoid tumor of the rectum. CT. Tumor does not extend beyond the bowel wall (PT2 N0).

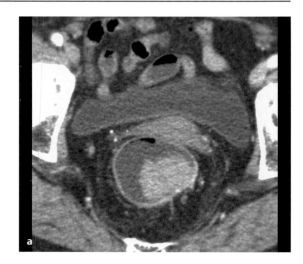

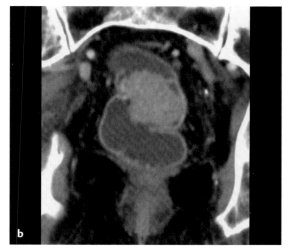

▶ **Findings on contrast enema**
Increasingly replaced by MRI • Irregular contour of the mucosa and narrowed lumen.

▶ **PET or PET/CT findings**
Most reliable modality for demonstrating extraintestinal recurrent tumors in scar tissue • Best demonstrates response to preoperative multimodal therapy.

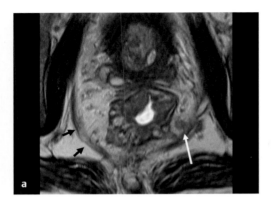

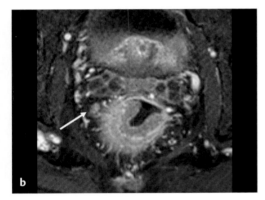

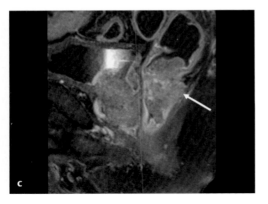

Fig. 8.15 a–c Carcinoma of the rectum extending beyond the bowel wall (T3 N1).
a T2-weighted MR image. Tumor extends into the mesorectal fatty tissue (black arrows: mesorectal fascia), enlarged lymph nodes (white arrow).
b T1-weighted MR image with fat suppression also clearly visualizes tumor growth beyond the bowel wall and an adjacent enlarged lymph node within the mesorectal fascia (arrow).
c Sagittal projection. Presacral tumor growth beyond the bowel wall (arrow).

Clinical Aspects

▶ **Typical presentation**
Remains asymptomatic for a long time ● Changes in bowel habits ● Blood in the stool.

▶ **Therapeutic options**
Resection with removal of the mesorectum ● Adjuvant radiation therapy and chemotherapy are indicated in advanced cases.

▶ **Course and prognosis**
Prognosis depends on the relationship of the tumor to the mesorectum ● Rate of local recurrence after curative resection is 30%.

▶ **What does the clinician want to know?**
Tumor stage ● Relationship of the tumor to the mesorectum.

Differential Diagnosis

Diverticulitis	– Thickening of a long segment of the bowel wall
	– Proved diverticula
	– Pericolic inflammation in adjacent fatty tissue
	– Thickening of the fascia
Ischemic colitis	– Long segment of thickened bowel wall
	– Reduced perfusion of the bowel wall
	– Occlusion or stenosis of arterial feeders
Ulcerative colitis	– Diffuse spread beginning in the rectum
	– Absence of haustration
Submucosal tumors (gastrointestinal stromal tumor, hemangioma)	– Eccentric narrowing of the lumen
Endometriosis	– External compression
	– Unilateral saw-tooth contour

Tips and Pitfalls

Insufficient filling of the colon with water on MRI is a common error ● Failing to match the imaging plane to the growth of the tumor is another.

Selected Literature

Beets-Tan RGH et al. Rectal cancer: review with emphasis on MR imaging. Radiology 2004; 232: 335–346

Brown G et al. Techniques and trouble-shooting in high spatial resolution thin slice MRI for rectal cancer. Br J Radiol 2005; 78: 245–251

Denecke T et al. Comparison of CT, MRI and FDG-PET in response prediction of patients with locally advanced rectal cancer after multimodal preoperative therapy: is there a benefit in using functional imaging? Eur Radiol 2005; 15: 1658–1666

Definition

Proliferation of ectopic endometrial tissue on or in the bowel wall.

▶ **Epidemiology**
Occurs in 15% of menstruating women and 30% of infertile women ● Usually occurs between the ages of 20 and 45 years ● The ectopic tissue is usually in the immediate vicinity of the uterus.

▶ **Etiology, pathophysiology, pathogenesis**
There are various hypotheses on the causes of extrauterine endometrial tissue ● Most likely it is the result of retrograde transport of endometrial tissue (retrograde menstruation) with implants in the pelvic organs and peritoneum ● Bowel involvement is rare, usually in the rectosigmoid (95% of all cases), appendix (10%), and ileum (5%) ● Further hematogenous and lymphatic spread is also possible ● As in the uterus, the ectopic tissue is influenced by hormones ● Serous inflammation and infiltration of the intestinal musculature can occur ● Obstruction of the affected bowel segment is possible ● *Rare complication:* Malignant degeneration.

Imaging Signs

▶ **Modality of choice**
Contrast enema, MRI.

▶ **Pathognomonic findings**
Submucosal polypoid mass (sawtooth impressions) ● Eccentric narrowing of the lumen ● Solid masses in the pelvis measuring 1–5 cm in diameter ● Endometrial cysts in the ovary.

▶ **MRI findings**
T1-weighted images show circumscribed, hypointense thickening of the bowel wall ● Eccentric narrowing of the lumen ● Small plaquelike serosal implants usually escape detection ● Solid, grossly fibrotic pelvic masses give an intermediate signal on T1-weighted images and a low signal on T2-weighted images ● Lesions enhance with contrast ● These nodules often show punctate hyperintensities on T1-weighted images apparently caused by hemorrhage.

▶ **Findings on contrast enema**
Submucosal polypoid nodules ● A sawtooth contour may be seen ● Eccentric narrowing of the lumen ● The structure of the mucosa is intact.

▶ **CT findings**
Circumscribed thickening of the bowel wall with eccentric narrowing of the lumen.

▶ **Endoscopic ultrasound findings**
The serosal implants and penetration of the bowel wall are well visualized ● Modality permits transmural guided biopsy.

▶ **Laparoscopy**
Often the diagnosis can only be made by direct inspection with guided biopsy.

Fig. 8.16 a–c Intestinal endometriosis. MR image.
a After the rectum is filled with water, findings include a hypointense polypoid mass obstructing the lumen.
b After contrast administration, the fat-suppressed image shows a uniformly enhancing mass. Findings also include apical strands of mucosal infiltration.
c The sagittal image shows a polypoid mass surrounded by a narrow halo of normal mucosa that appears slightly hyperintense.

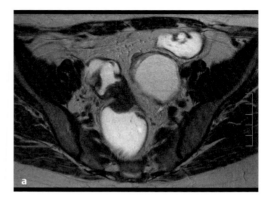

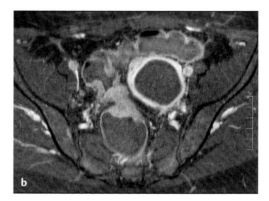

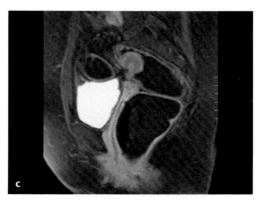

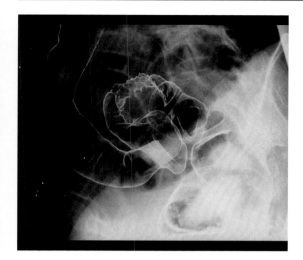

Fig. 8.17 Intestinal endometriosis. Double-contrast image of the rectum and sigmoid. Impression of the bowel lumen with a double contour and sawtooth irregularity due to infiltration of the mucosa.

Clinical Aspects

▶ **Typical presentation**

Symptoms are often absent or minimal ● Serosal implants create a sensation of tension in the pelvis ● Penetration into the bowel wall leads to constipation or diarrhea and painful bowel obstruction ● Penetration into the mucosa can lead to mucosal bleeding ● Symptoms vary with the menstrual cycle in only 40% of cases.

▶ **Therapeutic options**

Serosal implants are treated by laparoscopic laser ablation ● Penetration into the bowel wall with stenosis is treated by resection of the affected bowel segment.

▶ **Course and prognosis**

High rate of recurrence.

▶ **What does the clinician want to know?**

Exclude a malignant tumor or inflammatory bowel disease.

Differential Diagnosis

Submucosal tumors (gastrointestinal stromal tumor, hemangioma)	– Eccentric narrowing of the lumen – Usually large exophytic tumors – In advanced age
Colorectal carcinoma	– Irregular thickening of the wall – Concentric stenosis – In advanced age
Crohn disease and ulcerative colitis	– Concentric thickening of the bowel wall – Concentric stenosis – Absence of haustration
Diverticulitis	– Proved diverticula – Long segment of concentrically thickened bowel wall – Peridiverticulitis in the fatty tissue – Abscesses

Tips and Pitfalls

Insufficient filling of the rectosigmoid with water on cross-sectional modalities is a common error • Examination should be performed in the premenstrual phase.

Selected Literature

Bahr A et al. Endorectal ultrasonography in predicting rectal wall infiltration in patients with deep pelvic endometriosis: a modern tool for an ancient disease. Dis Colon Rectum 2006; 49: 869–875

Gordon RL et al. Double-contrast enema in pelvic endometriosis. AJR 1982; 138: 549–552

Siegelman ES et al. Solid pelvic masses caused by endometriosis: MR imaging features AJR 1994; 163: 357–361

Definition

Chronic suppurative infection in channels with an inner opening in the anal canal and orifice in the perianal region.

▶ **Epidemiology**

Prevalence is 10 : 100 000 • More common in men.

▶ **Etiology, pathophysiology, pathogenesis**

Over 90% of these lesions arise from inflammation of the proctodeal glands that usually lie between the sphincters and open at the level of the dentate line • Less common causes include ulcerative colitis, tuberculosis, and HIV infection • Fistulas in Crohn disease may be associated with inflammation of the proctodeal glands but may also arise from the anorectal canal independently of inflammation • 5–15% of fistulas exhibit a complex pattern of horseshoe-shaped fistulation and abscess formation in the ischiorectal region and above the levator muscle.

▶ **Park's classification:**

- *Superficial* (15%): The tract courses between the mucosa and internal sphincter to the perianal skin and does not cross the musculature.
- *Intersphincteric* (55%): The tract crosses the internal sphincter and courses between the internal and external sphincters.
- *Transsphincteric* (20%): The tract crosses the internal and external sphincters and courses into the ischiorectal fossa.
- *Suprasphincteric* (5%): The tract courses apically between the sphincters, curves above the puborectalis muscle, passes through the levator ani muscle, and then courses caudally into the ischiorectal fossa.
- *Extrasphincteral* (3%): The tract courses from the rectum to the perineum without any involvement of the anal canal or sphincteral musculature.

Imaging Signs

▶ **Modality of choice**

MRI, endosonography.

▶ **Pathognomonic findings**

Tubular structures in the anal canal coursing between or through the sphincters, above or below the levator ani muscle, or proximal to the sphincters • Abscesses (occasionally horseshoe-shaped) may or may not be present • Scarring is common.

▶ **MRI findings**

Modality of choice for imaging recurrent fistulas and Crohn disease • Does not require instrumentation and general anesthesia.

Musculature: The internal sphincter exhibits homogeneous structure on T2-weighted images and is hyperintense to the external sphincter • The external sphincter, puborectalis muscle, and levator sling are hypointense • On T1-weighted images, the muscles show no difference in signal intensity • The mucosa and internal sphincter enhance after contrast administration.

Fig. 8.18 a, b
Perianal abscess.
MR image, coronal.
a T1-weighted
image. Abscess in
the right ischiorec-
tal fossa, which sug-
gests spread of in-
flammation through
the sphincter.
b T2-weighted
image. The abscess
is hyperintense. The
fistula lies close to
the external sphinc-
ter at the level of
the proctodeal
glands.

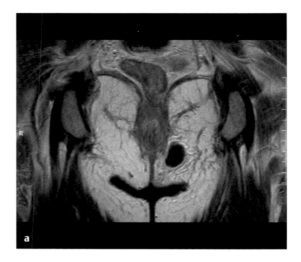

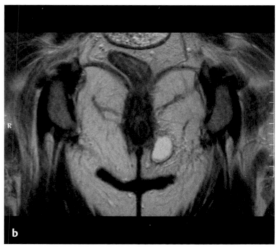

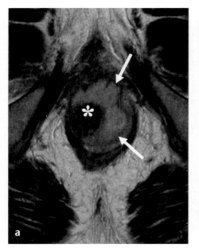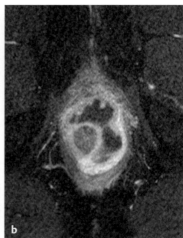

Fig. 8.19 a, b Perianal abscess. T2-weighted MR image, axial.
a Horseshoe-shaped abscess coursing between the sphincters (arrows).
The rectum is eccentric (asterisk).
b Contrast administration produces marked enhancement of the inflamed tissue
surrounding the abscess, which lies between the external and internal sphincter.

Fistulas: Fistulas without mucus appear as hypointense tubular structures on T2-weighted images • Mucus-filled fistulas show a hyperintense center surrounded by a hypointense ring • The inner opening can usually be identified (> 95 % of cases).

Abscesses: Fluid-filled hyperintense cavities • With fat suppression, the extent of inflammation can be readily evaluated • Contrast administration is helpful in certain cases to assess activity with greater precision.

► **Endosonographic findings**

Fistula tract is hypoechoic • Hyperechoic inclusions (gas) are occasionally present • The internal openings of the fistulas are well visualized (> 90 % of cases) • The depth of penetration is often insufficient for evaluating complex deep fistula systems • Modality of choice for simple fistulas.

► **Fistulographic findings**

Complete filling of the fistula tract is very unreliable and often painful • As it is often not possible to determine the relationship between the fistula tract and sphincter musculature, this modality has fallen from favor.

Clinical Aspects

▸ **Typical presentation**
  Anal and perianal pain • Secretion of pus, blood, mucus.
▸ **Therapeutic options**
  Surgical repair.
▸ **Course and prognosis**
  Recurrence is common, especially in complex fistula systems and where the extent of the fistula was not precisely determined preoperatively.
▸ **What does the clinician want to know?**
  Extent of fistulas and abscesses.

Differential Diagnosis

Hidradenitis	– Anogenital and inguinal region
	– Patchy skin disorder with fistulation and abscesses
	– Thickening of the skin and subcutaneous tissue
Crohn Disease	– Fistulas often show no relationship to the proctodeal glands
	– Diarrhea
	– Known disorder with involvement of the colon
Veins and hemorrhoids	– Tortuous course
	– Thin walled
	– Findings on inspection and palpation
Pilonidal sinus	– No relationship to the intersphincteric fissure

Tips and Pitfalls

Incorrect imaging axis on MRI.

Selected Literature

Beets-Tan RGH et al. Preoperative MR imaging of anal fistulas: does it really help the surgeon. Radiology 2001; 218: 75–84

Buchanan GN et al. Clinical examination, endosonography, and MR imaging in preoperative assessment of fistulo in ano: comparison with outcome-based reference standard. Radiology 2004; 233: 674–681

Horsthuis K et al. MRI of perianal Crohn's disease. AJR 2004; 183: 1309–1315

Definition

Developmental abnormality with a presacral cystic mass that tends to become infected and has potential for malignant degeneration.

▶ **Epidemiology**
This rare lesion is the most common developmental anomaly in the retrorectal space • Occurs primarily in middle-aged women.

▶ **Etiology, pathophysiology, pathogenesis**
Developmental anomaly involving a tailgut cyst • *Two types:* Cystic hamartomas and duplication cysts • There is no communication with the rectum.

Imaging Signs

▶ **Modality of choice**
MRI, CT.

▶ **Pathognomonic findings**
Well-demarcated cystic mass • Single cyst or multiple cysts with thin walls • Irregular thickening of the cyst wall with contrast enhancement suggests malignant degeneration • Bone defects in the sacrum are rare.

▶ **MRI findings**
Hypointense on T1-weighted images • Homogeneously hyperintense on T2-weighted images • Cysts with mucinous contents, hemorrhage, or fatty components (dermoid cysts) appear hyperintense on T1-weighted images.

▶ **CT findings**
Smoothly marginated cystic mass • Contents are isodense to water or soft tissue • Septa are less clearly identifiable.

▶ **Ultrasound findings**
Cysts may contain internal echoes, especially in infections.

Clinical Aspects

▶ **Typical presentation**
Often asymptomatic • There may be a mass effect • Constipation • Sensation of fullness in the rectum • Pain on defecation • Pain in the lower abdomen • Dysuria • Rectal examination reveals a palpable tumor.

▶ **Therapeutic options**
Surgical removal is usually indicated due to the risk of inflammation and malignant degeneration • Patients not treated surgically require regular follow-up.

▶ **Course and prognosis**
Complications: Infection with fistulation (in 30–50% of cases) • Bleeding • Malignant degeneration (10%).

▶ **What does the clinician want to know?**
Are there signs of inflammation or malignant degeneration? • Extent and relationship to adjacent structures • Reliably exclude a tumor.

Fig. 8.20 a, b
Retrorectal cystic hamartoma. CT. Unilocular retrorectal cyst directly adjacent to the rectum.

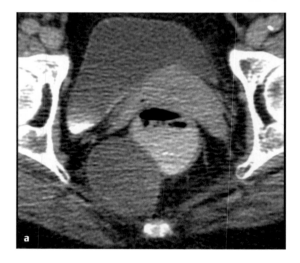

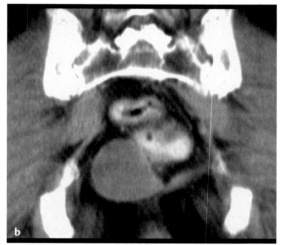

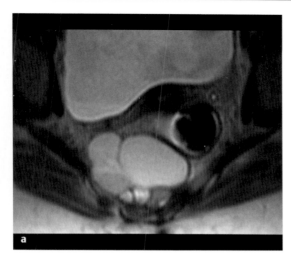

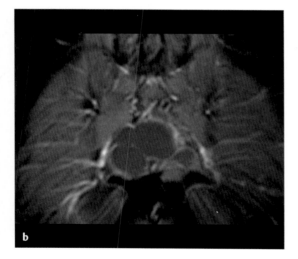

Fig. 8.21 a, b
Retrorectal cystic hamartoma. MR image. Multiloculated retrorectal cyst.
a T2-weighted image.
b T1-weighted image after intravenous contrast administration.

Differential Diagnosis

Cystic teratoma	– In 90% of cases, this condition is diagnosed in newborns (girls) – Cross-sectional studies show an inhomogeneous lesion with solid and cystic components – Half of all lesions contain fat or calcifications
Anterior sacral meningocele	– Herniation of the dural sac through the bony defect in partial sacral agenesis
Cystic lymphangioma	– Usually in children – Well-demarcated, thin-walled multicystic mass
Abscess	– Most often postoperative or in inflammation such as appendicitis or Crohn disease
Leiomyosarcoma of the rectum	– Thickening of the rectal wall – More common in men
Chordoma of the sacrum	– Bony destruction of the sacrum – Primarily solid tumor

Tips and Pitfalls

Because it is rare, this lesion is often diagnosed late or incorrectly, leading to incorrect treatment such as drainage.

Selected Literature

Dahan H et al. Retrorectal developmental cysts in adults: clinical and radiologic-histopathologic review, differential diagnosis, and treatment. RadioGraphics 2001; 21: 575–584

Johnson AR et al. Tailgut cyst: diagnosis with CT and sonography. AJR 1986; 147: 1309–1311

Yang DM et al. Tailgut cyst: MRI evaluation. AJR 2005; 184: 1519–1523

Definition

▶ **Epidemiology**
Most common malignant disorder of the peritoneum.
▶ **Etiology, pathophysiology, pathogenesis**
Most common primary tumors—ovary, stomach, colon, breast, pancreas, lung, sarcomas, lymphomas.
Pseudomyxoma peritonei: Rare form with gelatinous implants in the peritoneal space ● 75% of cases involve women aged 45–75 years ● Primary tumors in the appendix and ovary.

Imaging Signs

▶ **Modality of choice**
CT ● Ultrasound (with ascites).
▶ **Pathognomonic findings**
Ascites, occasionally sparing the lesser pelvis ● Peritoneal nodules that variably enhance ● Confluent nodules in the omentum ("omental cake" pattern) ● Adhesions and abnormal strands in the mesentery ● Bowel loops no longer float on the surface ● Encased bowel loops that are dilated proximal to the stenosis.
▶ **CT findings**
The extent of the ascites, peritoneal implants, and omental involvement are best evaluated on CT ● Stenoses of the small bowel and colon are most readily detectable after oral and/or rectal administration of diluted contrast agent ● Metastases in the liver, lungs, bone, and lymph nodes can be evaluated.
▶ **MRI findings**
Ascites is hypointense on T1-weighted images ● Peritoneal implants and omental involvement exhibit medium signal intensity ● Ascites is hyperintense and metastases exhibit medium signal intensity on T2-weighted images ● Contrast enhancement in the peritoneum.
▶ **Ultrasound findings**
Where ascites is present, findings include metastases in the omentum and nodular pathology on the peritoneum ● In the absence of ascites, examination provides limited diagnostic information.

Fig. 9.1 a, b
Pseudomyxoma peritonei. CT.
a Between the ascites and the shortened bowel loop there is a slightly denser layer of gelatinous material (arrows).
b The tumorous masses have led to bizarre deformation of the contour of the liver.

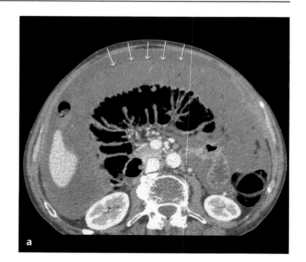

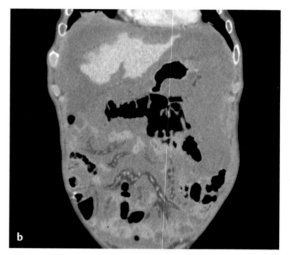

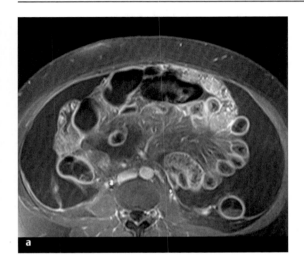

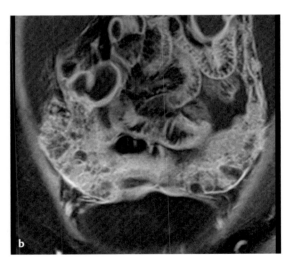

Fig. 9.2 a, b Peritoneal carcinomatosis in ovarian carcinoma. MR image (axial). (**a**) and coronal (**b**) T1-weighted images after intravenous administration of gadolinium. Shortened mesentery loops and omental tumor masses ("omental cake") in the anterior middle and lower abdomen.

Clinical Aspects

▶ **Typical presentation**
Usually in advanced tumor • Usually ascites, weight loss, and abdominal pain •
May be the first clinical sign in ovarian carcinoma.

▶ **Therapeutic options**
Surgical intervention is rarely indicated • Intraperitoneal chemotherapy.

▶ **Course and prognosis**
Prognosis is usually very poor • Most patients live less than 1 month, 25% survive 3 months, and only 10% survive 6 months • One exception is ovarian carcinoma, where surgical debulking and chemotherapy can significantly prolong
life • Recurrent and increasing bowel obstruction.

▶ **What does the clinician want to know?**
Cause of ascites • What is the risk of bowel obstruction?

Differential Diagnosis

Peritonitis	– Significant contrast enhancement in the peritoneum
	– Bowel loops float on the ascites
	– No tumor nodules
Peritoneal mesothelioma	– Tumor growth over a broad area on the peritoneum
	– Often the tumor infiltrates into the outer layers of the abdominal wall
	– Common in patients with a history of years of exposure to asbestos
Cirrhosis of the liver	– Altered size, shaped, and structure of the liver
	– Signs of portal hypertension (varices)
	– Bowel loops float on the ascites
Abdominal lipomatosis	– On CT isodense and on MRI isointense to fat

Tips and Pitfalls

Can be misinterpreted as ascites in portal hypertension • Tumor nodules can be
quite discrete.

Selected Literature

Hanbidge AE et al. US of the peritoneum. RadioGraphics 2003; 23: 663–684
Raptopoulos V et al. Peritoneal carcinomatosis. Eur Radiol 2001; 11: 2195–2206
Sulkin TV et al. CT in pseudomyxoma peritonei: a review of 17 cases. Clin Radiol 2002; 57:
    608–613

Page numbers in *italics* refer to
illustrations.

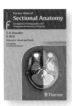

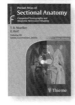
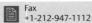

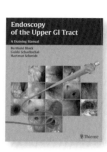
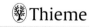